Pocket
for Nurs

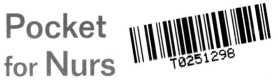

T0251298

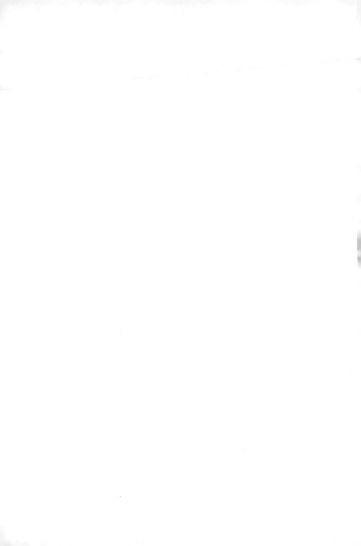

Pocket ECGs
for Nurses

Andrew R. Houghton
MA (Oxon) DM FRCP (London & Glasgow),
Consultant Cardiologist,
Grantham and District Hospital,
Grantham, UK

Alun Roebuck
Lincolnshire Heart Centre,
Lincoln County Hospital, UK

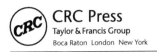

CRC Press
Taylor & Francis Group
Boca Raton London New York

CRC Press is an imprint of the
Taylor & Francis Group, an **informa** business

CRC Press
Taylor & Francis Group
6000 Broken Sound Parkway NW, Suite 300
Boca Raton, FL 33487-2742

© 2016 by Taylor & Francis Group, LLC
CRC Press is an imprint of Taylor & Francis Group, an Informa business

No claim to original U.S. Government works

Printed on acid-free paper
Version Date: 20151022

International Standard Book Number-13: 978-1-4987-0593-6 (Paperback)

Contents

Preface ix
Acknowledgements xi

1 The basics of the heartbeat 1
The heart chambers 1
The heart's myocytes 5
Anatomy of the electrical system 7
Further reading 10

2 The basics of the ECG 11
ECG leads 11
The names of the ECG waves 14
Normal values 16
QRS ('cardiac') axis 19
Abnormal cardiac axis 23
Further reading 23

3 How to record a 12-lead ECG 25
Initial preparations 25
Skin preparation 26
Electrode placement 27
Special electrode positions 32
Recording the 12-lead ECG 34
After making the recording 38
Further reading 38

4 How to read a 12-lead ECG 41
Patient data 41
Clinical data 42
Technical data 42

ECG fundamentals 43
ECG details 43
Clinical summary 44
Further reading 45

5 Heart rate: Bradycardia and tachycardia 47
Method 1: Counting large squares 48
Method 2: Counting small squares 48
Method 3: Counting QRS complexes 50
P wave rate 52
Bradycardia and tachycardia 52
Further reading 62

6 An approach to heart rhythms 63
Identifying the cardiac rhythm 65
Determining the cardiac rhythm 76
Further reading 77

7 Supraventricular rhythms 79
Sinus rhythm 79
Sinus arrhythmia 79
Sinus bradycardia 82
Sinus tachycardia 84
Sick sinus syndrome 84
Atrial ectopic beats 86
Atrial fibrillation 88
Atrial flutter 91
Atrial tachycardia 94
AV re-entry tachycardia 94
AV nodal re-entry tachycardia 103
Further reading 105

8 Ventricular rhythms 107
Ventricular ectopic beats 107

Monomorphic ventricular tachycardia — 114
Polymorphic ventricular tachycardia — 124
Ventricular fibrillation — 127
Further reading — 128

9 Conduction problems and types of block — 129
Conduction problems at the SA node — 129
Conduction problems at the AV node — 130
Block at the bundle branches — 136
Block at the fascicles — 144
Escape rhythms — 146
Further reading — 147

10 QRS complexes and left ventricular hypertrophy — 149
Q wave — 149
Tall QRS complexes — 151
Small QRS complexes — 156
Broad QRS complexes — 159
Further reading — 163

11 ST segment elevation and depression — 165
Assessing the ST segment — 165
ST segment elevation — 170
ST segment depression — 181
Further reading — 186

12 T wave changes — 187
Tall upright T waves — 187
Small T waves — 190
Inverted T waves — 193
Further reading — 197

13 QT interval prolongation — 199
What is the QT interval? — 199
Measuring the QT interval — 200

'Correcting' the QT interval   202
What is a normal QTc interval?   205
Risks of a long QT interval   207
Causes of a long QT interval   209
Treatment of a long QT interval   212
Further reading   212

14 Bedside and ambulatory monitoring   **213**
Inpatient ECG monitoring   213
Outpatient ECG monitoring   215
The future of ECG monitoring   219
Further reading   220

15 Summary of key points   **221**
Basics of the heartbeat   221
Basics of the ECG   222
How to record a 12-lead ECG   224
How to read a 12-lead ECG   225
Heart rate: Tachycardia and bradycardia   226
Approach to heart rhythms   227
Supraventricular rhythms   228
Ventricular rhythms   228
Conduction problems and types of block   229
QRS complexes and left ventricular hypertrophy   230
ST segment elevation and depression   231
T wave changes   232
QT interval prolongation   232
Bedside and ambulatory monitoring   233

Appendix A: ECG resources   235
Appendix B: Help with the next edition   239
Index   241

Preface

The ECG is one of the most commonly used investigations in contemporary medicine. Interpretation of the ECG can appear daunting, but it is actually relatively straightforward as long as a systematic approach is taken.

In *Pocket ECGs for Nurses*, we aim to provide nursing colleagues with a detailed yet readable introduction to ECG interpretation, supplemented by clinical information about how to act upon your findings.

We guide you through the basics of cardiac anatomy and physiology and how they relate to the ECG. We provide information on how to perform a high-quality ECG recording and how to approach its interpretation. We then guide you step by step through heart rhythms and how to make sense of common ECG abnormalities. We end the book with a guide to bedside and ambulatory monitoring and a useful summary of each chapter.

We hope that you find *Pocket ECGs for Nurses* a valuable guide in learning how to perform and read an ECG and a useful reference for everyday practice.

Andrew R. Houghton
Alun Roebuck

Acknowledgements

We thank everyone who gave us suggestions and constructive criticism during the preparation of *Pocket ECGs for Nurses*. We are particularly grateful to all those who have allowed us to use ECGs from their collections. We are also grateful to the Resuscitation Council (UK) for their permission to reproduce algorithms from their adult advanced life support guidelines (2015).

Finally, we also like to express our gratitude to Naomi Wilkinson and the rest of the publishing team at CRC Press for their encouragement, guidance and support during this project.

Chapter 1

The basics of the heartbeat

The heart is a cone-shaped muscular organ located slightly to the left of the sternum, between the lungs and in front of the spine. The top of the heart (known as its 'base') is approximately in line with the second rib, and the tip of the cone (known as its 'apex') points down and rests on the diaphragm (Figure 1.1).

The heart chambers

The heart consists of four chambers: the left and right atria, and the left and right ventricles. Contraction of the ventricles is called *systole*, and during systole blood is pumped to the lungs (by the right ventricle) and around the body (by the left ventricle). The period in between ventricular contractions is called *diastole*, and during

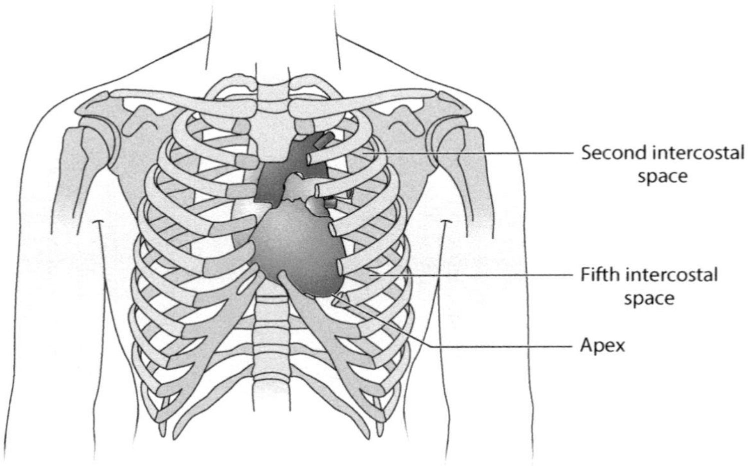

Figure 1.1 Location of the heart within the chest.

Second intercostal space

Fifth intercostal space

Apex

this time the ventricles fill with blood ready for the next heartbeat (Figure 1.2).

The atria are situated above the ventricles and contract at the end of diastole, just before the ventricles contract in systole. Most (85%) of the filling of the ventricles during diastole occurs 'passively' – that is to say, blood flows from the atria to the ventricles down a 'pressure gradient' with no active involvement by the heart itself. However, at the end of diastole, the atria contract and squeeze some more blood into the ventricles. This 'atrial kick' accounts for 15% of ventricular filling. If patients lose this atrial kick (for instance, when they develop atrial fibrillation), then the ventricles no longer fill quite as effectively and this can cause symptoms of breathlessness and fatigue.

The right ventricle is less muscular than the left ventricle because it only has to pump blood to the lungs (where it becomes oxygenated). The left ventricle is much more muscular than the right ventricle as it has to pump blood around the rest of the body. The heart chambers are separated by valves (Figure 1.3), the purpose of which is to stop blood flowing back the wrong way during the cardiac cycle.

The normal resting heart rate is between 60 and 100 beats/min, and with each beat the heart pumps about 70 ml of blood (this is known as the *stroke volume*). Therefore the heart will beat approximately 100,000 times a day pumping approximately 7,000 L of blood.

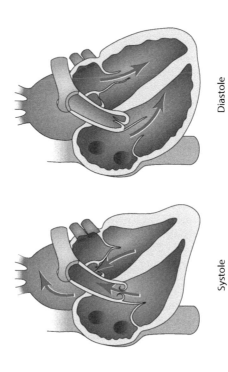

Systole   Diastole

Figure 1.2 Ventricular systole (contraction) and diastole (relaxation).

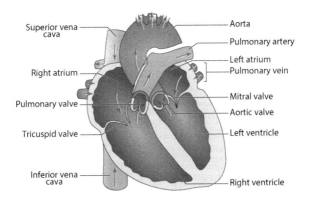

Figure 1.3 Anatomy of the heart and its major vessels.

The heart's myocytes

The heart is made up of highly specialized cardiac muscle comprising myocardial cells (*myocytes*). Myocytes are essentially contractile but are capable of generating and transmitting electrical activity. Myocytes are electrically interconnected, so once one myocyte is activated ('depolarized'), a wave of depolarization spreads rapidly to adjacent cells. Myocardial cells are capable of being

- *Pacemaker cells*: These are found primarily in the sinoatrial (SA) node and produce a spontaneous electrical discharge that acts as the heart's natural pacemaker

- *Conducting cells*: These conduct impulses between different areas of the heart, and are found in the atrioventricular (AV) node, the bundle of His and bundle branches, and the Purkinje fibres
- *Contractile cells*: These form the main cell type in the atria and ventricles.

The brain tells the heart's natural pacemaker how quickly to beat via two branches of the autonomic nervous system: the *sympathetic* branch (sometimes known as adrenergic) and the *parasympathetic* branch (sometimes known as cholinergic). The sympathetic branch acts as the heart's accelerator and increases the heart rate, while the parasympathetic branch serves as the brakes, slowing the heart.

All myocytes are self-excitable with their own intrinsic contractile rhythm. Cardiac cells in the SA node generate impulses at a rate of about 60–100/min, a slightly faster rate than cells elsewhere, such as the AV node (typically 40–60/min) or the ventricular conducting system (30–40/min), so the SA node acts as the heart's pacemaker, dictating the rate and timing of action potentials that trigger cardiac contraction, overriding the potential of other cells to generate impulses. However, should the SA node fail, or an impulse not reach the ventricles, cardiac contraction may be initiated by these secondary sites – these are called 'escape rhythms'.

THE CARDIAC ACTION POTENTIAL

Cardiac myocytes undergo cycles of depolarization and repolarization. Cells are considered polarized when no electrical activity is taking place. Membranes in the cardiac myocyte separate different concentrations of ions (salts) such as sodium, potassium, chloride and magnesium. When the cell is stimulated, ions cross the membrane and cause the cell to depolarize. Once a cell is fully depolarized, it attempts to return to its resting state: this is known as repolarization. The depolarization–repolarization cycle is made up of five phases (Figure 1.4):

- **Phase 0** – The cell receives an impulse from the neighbouring cell and is depolarized.
- **Phase 1** – Early rapid repolarization.
- **Phase 2** – Late slow repolarization.
- **Phase 3** – Absolute refractory period (at this time no stimulus can excite the cell).
- **Phase 4** – The resting phase (by the end of phase 4 the cell is ready to do it all over again).

Anatomy of the electrical system

In order for the heart to beat efficiently, the chambers need to contract in the correct sequence. If they contract out of sequence or in a disorganized manner (*dyssynchrony*) the heart becomes less efficient and the patient may develop symptoms that impact on their quality of life. The contraction of the heart chambers and the coordination of its timing are controlled by the heart's electrical system (Figure 1.5).

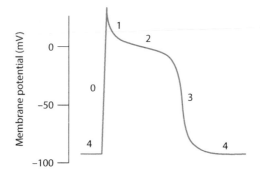

Figure 1.4 The cardiac action potential. Phases 0–4 are marked.

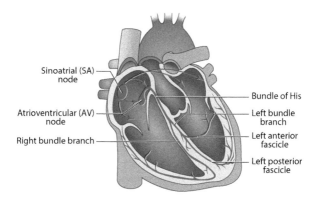

Figure 1.5 The cardiac conduction system.

Sinoatrial node

The SA node is located in the right atrium near its junction with the superior vena cava. The SA node acts as the pacemaker of the heart. It generates electrical impulses that are transmitted to all parts of the heart. The rate at which the SA node generates impulses depends on the demands from the body. A normal resting heart rate for an adult is between 60 and 100 beats/min but this can rise to 150 beats/min or more with energetic physical exertion.

Once an impulse leaves the SA node, it travels across the atria from myocyte to myocyte, causing the atria to depolarize and contract. This wavefront of depolarization then reaches the AV node to initiate the next phase of cardiac conduction.

Atrioventricular node

The AV node is located between the septal leaflet of tricuspid valve, the coronary sinus and the inter-atrial septum. The role of the AV node is to slow down the electrical impulse before transmitting it on to the ventricles – this allows time for the atria to contract before the ventricles contract.

Bundle of His

Once an impulse has passed through the AV node, it enters the bundle of His, which rapidly transmits the impulse on to the left and right bundle branches.

Bundle branches

The left and right bundle branches act as high-speed pathways that rapidly transmit the impulse to the left and right ventricles. The left bundle branch divides into two smaller branches, called the anterior and posterior fascicles.

Purkinje fibres

The Purkinje fibres are fine pathways at the end of the bundle branches that quickly distribute the electrical impulse throughout the ventricles, ensuring that ventricular depolarization (and contraction) occur rapidly.

Further reading

Cabrera JA, Sánchez-Quintana D. Cardiac anatomy: What the electrophysiologist needs to know. *Heart* 2013; **99**: 417–431.

Chockalingam P, Wilde A. The multifaceted cardiac sodium channel and its clinical implications. *Heart* 2012; **98**: 1318–1324.

Chapter 2

The basics of the ECG

An electrocardiogram (ECG) is a recording of the electrical activity of the heart over a period of time (in practice, a standard 12-lead ECG is typically recorded over a period of 10 s). The ECG is recorded by placing electrodes in standardized positions on the limbs and chest wall. These electrodes record the small electrical changes that come from the heart when it depolarizes.

ECG leads

To understand the ECG, one of the most important concepts to grasp is that of the 'lead'. This is a term you will often see, and it does *not* refer to the wires that connect the patient to the ECG machine (which we will always refer to as 'electrodes' to avoid confusion).

In short, 'leads' are different *viewpoints* of the heart's electrical activity. An ECG machine uses the information it collects via its four limb and six chest electrodes to compile a comprehensive picture of the electrical activity in the heart as observed from 12 different viewpoints (Figure 2.1)

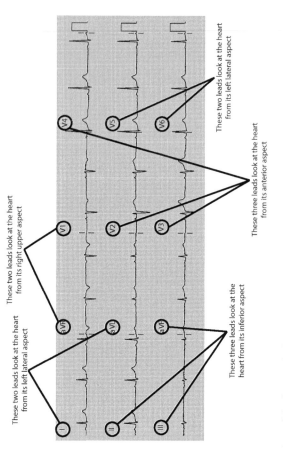

Figure 2.1 The standard 12-lead ECG and the 'view' from each lead.

and this set of 12 views or leads gives the 12-lead ECG its name. Having a number of different views of the heart is very useful – it allows us to localize the region of the heart affected by a myocardial infarction, for instance, and can also be very useful in the diagnosis of arrhythmias.

Each lead is given a name and its position on a 12-lead ECG is usually standardized to make pattern recognition easier. So what viewpoint does each lead have of the heart? Information from the four limb electrodes is used by the ECG machine to create the six limb leads (I, II, III, aVR, aVL and aVF). Each limb lead 'looks' at the heart from the side (the frontal or 'coronal' plane), and the view that each lead has of the heart in this plane depends on the lead in question (Figure 2.2).

As you can see from Figure 2.2, lead aVR looks at the heart from the approximate viewpoint of the patient's right shoulder, whereas leads I and aVL have a left lateral view of the heart, and leads II, III and aVF look at the inferior surface of the heart.

The six chest leads (V1–V6) look at the heart in a horizontal ('transverse') plane from the front and around the side of the chest (Figure 2.3). The region of myocardium surveyed by each lead therefore varies according to its vantage point – leads V3–V4 have an anterior view, for example, whereas leads V5–V6 have a lateral view.

Once you know the view each lead has of the heart, you can tell if the electrical impulses in the heart are flowing towards that lead or away from it. This is simple to work out, because electrical current flowing towards a lead produces an upward (positive) deflection on the ECG, whereas current flowing

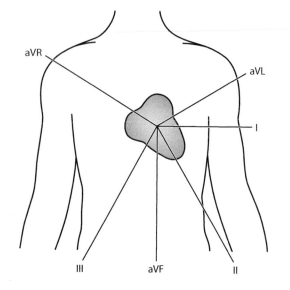

Figure 2.2 The viewpoint each limb lead has of the heart.
The limb leads look at the heart in the frontal ('coronal') plane,
and each limb lead looks at the heart from a different angle.

The names of the ECG waves

As discussed in Chapter 1, once the sinoatrial (SA) node
initiates an electrical impulse, a wave of electrical activity
cascades through the heart causing its various chambers to
depolarize (and contract). This is followed by repolarization,
when the chambers 'recharge' and get ready for the next
heartbeat.

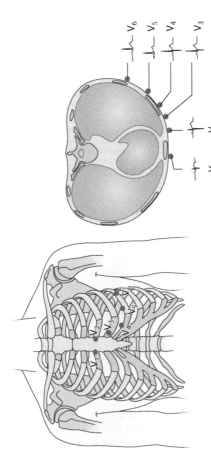

Figure 2.3 The viewpoint each chest lead has of the heart. Each chest lead looks at the heart from a different viewpoint in the horizontal ('transverse') plane.

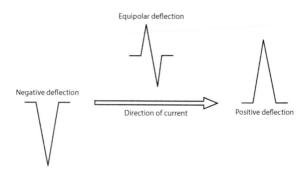

Figure 2.4 The direction of an ECG deflection depends upon the direction of the current. Flow towards a lead produces a positive deflection, flow away from a lead produces a negative deflection and flow perpendicular to a lead produces a positive then a negative (equipolar or isoelectric) deflection.

This wave of depolarization and repolarization generates deflections on the ECG as it passes through the heart (Figure 2.5), and each component has its own unique name and clinical significance, as detailed in Table 2.1.

Normal values

In addition to understanding the waves and intervals of the ECG and what they correspond to, the nurse also needs to be aware of the range of normal values for various measurements that can be taken from the ECG.

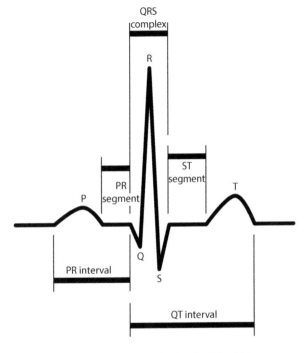

Figure 2.5 The principal waves and intervals of the ECG.

A *resting heart rate* of between 60 and 100 beats/min is the normal range for an adult:
- Bradycardia is a heart rate of less than 60 beats/min
- Tachycardia is a heart rate of greater than 100 beats/min.

Table 2.1 The waves and intervals of the ECG and the events they correspond to

ECG event	Cardiac event
P wave	Atrial depolarization
PR interval	Start of atrial depolarization to start of ventricular depolarization
QRS complex	Ventricular depolarization
ST segment	Pause in ventricular electrical activity before repolarization
T wave	Ventricular repolarization
QT interval	Total time taken by ventricular depolarization and repolarization
U wave	Uncertain – possibly: • Interventricular septal repolarization • Slow ventricular repolarization

Note: Depolarization of the SA and AV nodes are important events but do not, in themselves, produce a detectable wave on a standard ECG.

The *PR interval* is measured from the beginning of the P wave to the beginning of the QRS complex (Figure 2.5) and reflects the time taken for the electrical impulse to travel from the SA node to the atrioventricular (AV) node (including atrial depolarization):

• Short PR interval is <120 ms.
• Normal PR interval is 120–200 ms.
• Long PR interval is >200 ms.

The *QRS duration* represents ventricular depolarization and is measured from the beginning of the Q wave to the end of the S wave, and this usually occurs in less than 120 ms. Therefore

- Normal QRS duration is <120 ms.
- Prolonged QRS duration ('broad QRS') is >120 ms.

The *QT interval* measures the total time for activation of the ventricles and recovery to the normal resting state and is measured from the beginning of the QRS complex to the end of the T wave. The measurement and 'correction' of the QT interval, together with the normal values, are discussed in Chapter 13.

QRS ('cardiac') axis

Many people find the concept of the QRS axis difficult. Hence, it is often not applied as widely as it should be. However, the axis is actually fairly straightforward. Indeed, deciding whether the QRS axis is normal can be summarized in one rule:

A QUICK RULE FOR ASSESSING THE AXIS

If the QRS complexes are predominantly positive in leads I and II, the QRS axis is normal.

The QRS axis is an indicator of the general direction that the wave of depolarization takes as it flows through the ventricles – in other words, the overall vector of ventricular depolarization. If you think just about the general direction of electrical current as it flows through

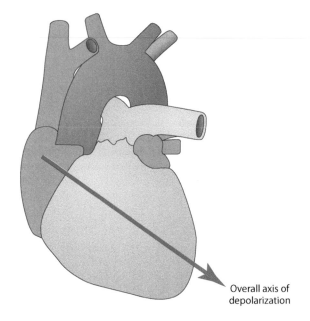

Figure 2.6 The overall direction of depolarization of the ventricles (QRS or 'cardiac' axis).

the ventricles, it starts at the base of the heart and flows towards the apex (Figure 2.6).

The QRS axis is therefore conventionally referred to as the angle, measured in degrees, of the direction of electrical current flowing through the ventricles. The reference, or zero, point is taken as a horizontal line 'looking' at the heart

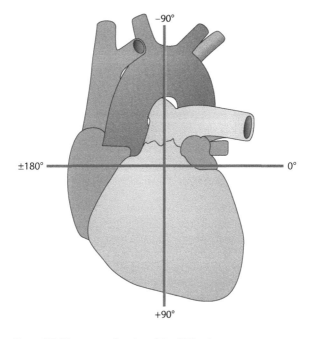

Figure 2.7 **The range of angles of the QRS axis.**

below the line, the angle is expressed as a positive number; above the line, as a negative number. Thus, the axis can be either +1° to +180° or −1° to −180°.

- A normal cardiac axis lies between −30° and +90°.
- Left axis deviation lies between −30° and −90°.
- Right axis deviation lies between +90° and +180°.

	Normal axis	Left axis deviation	Right axis deviation	Extreme right axis deviation
Lead I	∧	∧	∨	∨
Lead II	∧	∨	∧	∨

Figure 2.8 The quick 'eyeball' method of assessing QRS axis using leads I and II.

There are several ways of working out QRS axis (some more complicated than others). We have tried to make this book as useful as possible to nonspecialists and hence we will only describe the easiest method of 'eyeball' inspection. While easy to remember, this technique is not as sensitive as some of the other methods (but in everyday clinical practice this makes little difference) (Figure 2.8).

To 'eyeball' the QRS axis, take a look at the QRS complexes in leads I and II. Are the QRS complexes in these leads predominantly positive ('upright') or negative ('downward pointing')?

- A positive QRS complex in both leads I and II means the *axis is normal.*
- A positive QRS complex in lead I and a negative QRS complex in lead II mean there is *left axis deviation.*
- A negative QRS complex in lead I and a positive QRS

- A negative QRS complex in lead I and a negative QRS complex in lead II mean there is *extreme right axis deviation*.

Abnormal cardiac axis

If the axis is abnormal, the next question is why?

Causes of left axis deviation

- Left anterior fascicular block
- Left bundle branch block
- Secondary to a paced rhythm
- Inferior myocardial infarction
- Wolff–Parkinson–White (WPW) syndrome
- Ventricular tachycardia

Causes of right axis deviation

- Left posterior fascicular block
- Right ventricular hypertrophy
- Anterolateral myocardial infarction
- WPW syndrome
- Dextrocardia

Further reading

Hurst JW. Naming of the waves in the ECG, with a brief account of their genesis. *Circulation* 1998; **98**: 1937–1942.

Meek S, Morri F. ABC of clinical electrocardiography: Introduction. I—Leads, rate, rhythm, and cardiac axis. *Br Med J* 2002; **324**: 415–418.

Chapter 3

How to record a 12-lead ECG

Recording a high-quality ECG is essential to ensure that interpretation of the ECG is correct. Errors that can occur in ECG recording include poor electrode contact and incorrect electrode positioning, which can lead to misinterpretation of the ECG and misdiagnosis.

This guide to performing a standard 12-lead ECG recording is based upon the current clinical guidelines of the Society for Cardiological Science and Technology in the United Kingdom (see *Further Reading*). Anyone performing a 12-lead ECG recording should have received appropriate training and been assessed in their skills by a competent practitioner.

Initial preparations

Before making a 12-lead ECG recording, check that the ECG machine is safe to use and has been cleaned appropriately. Before you start, ensure you have an adequate supply of

- Recording paper
- Skin preparation equipment
- Electrodes

Introduce yourself to the patient and confirm their identity. Explain what you plan to do and why, and ensure that they consent to undergo the ECG recording.

The 12-lead ECG should be recorded with the patient lying supine on a couch or bed, in a warm environment, while ensuring that the patient is comfortable and able to relax. This is not only important for patient dignity, but also helps to ensure a high-quality recording with minimal artefact.

Skin preparation

In order to apply the electrodes, the patient's skin needs to be exposed across the chest, the arms and the lower legs. Ensure that you follow your local chaperone policy, and offer the patient a gown to cover any exposed areas once the electrodes are applied.

To optimize electrode contact with the patient's skin and reduce 'noise', consider the following tips.

Removal of chest hair

It may be necessary to remove chest hair in the areas where the electrodes are to be applied. Ensure the patient consents to this before you start. Carry a supply of disposable razors with your ECG machine for this purpose.

Light abrasion

Exfoliation of the skin using light abrasion can help improve electrode contact. This can be achieved using specially manufactured abrasive tape or by using a
paper towel

Skin cleansing

An alcohol wipe helps to remove grease from the surface
of the skin, although this may be better avoided if patients
have fragile or broken skin.

Electrode placement

Correct placement of ECG electrodes is essential to
ensure that the 12-lead ECG can be interpreted correctly.
A standard 12-lead ECG consists of

- Three bipolar limb leads (I, II and III)
- Three augmented limb leads (aVR, aVL and aVF)
- Six chest (or 'precordial') leads (V1–V6)

As we saw in Chapter 2, these 12 leads are generated using
10 ECG electrodes, four of which are applied to the limbs and six
to the chest. The ECG electrodes are colour-coded to aid correct
placement; in Europe, the following colour codes are used:

Right arm	Red
Left arm	Yellow
Right leg	Black
Left leg	Green
Chest V1	White/red
Chest V2	White/yellow
Chest V3	White/green
Chest V4	White/brown
Chest V5	White/black
Chest V6	White/violet

To help you in placing the limb electrodes, remember the mnemonic 'Ride Your Green Bike'. Start by attaching the red ('Ride') electrode on the patient's right arm, then move around the patient's torso clockwise, attaching the yellow ('Your') electrode on the left arm, then the green ('Green') electrode on the left leg and finally the black ('Bike') electrode on the right leg.

ELECTRODE MISPLACEMENT

Electrode misplacement is a common occurrence, reported in 0.4% of ECGs recorded in the cardiac outpatient clinic and 4.0% of ECGs recorded in the intensive care unit. Incorrect positioning of the electrodes can have major effects on the appearance of the ECG, and can lead to misdiagnosis and inappropriate tests or treatment.

Placement of the limb electrodes

Attach the four limb electrodes to the arms and legs just proximal to the wrist and ankle (Figure 3.1). If the electrodes have to be placed in a more proximal position on the limb (e.g. if the patient has leg ulcers or a previous amputation), note this on the ECG recording. Placing the limb electrodes more proximally on the limbs can alter the appearance of the ECG and it is therefore important that the person interpreting the recording is aware that an atypical electrode position has been used.

Placement of the chest (precordial) electrodes

Position the six chest electrodes on the chest wall as shown in Figure 3.2. Common errors include placing electrodes

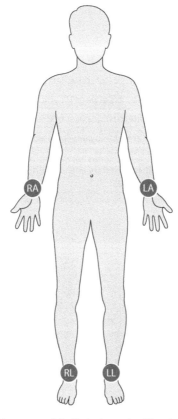

Figure 3.1 Placement of the limb electrodes. The electrodes are placed on the right arm (RA), left arm (LA), right leg (RL)

V1 and V2 too high and V5 and V6 too low. The correct locations are as follows:

Chest V1	4th intercostal space, right sternal edge
Chest V2	4th intercostal space, left sternal edge
Chest V3	Midway in between V2 and V4
Chest V4	5th intercostal space, mid-clavicular line
Chest V5	Left anterior axillary line, same horizontal level as V4
Chest V6	Left mid-axillary line, same horizontal level as V4 and V5

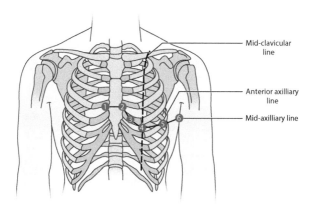

Figure 2.2 Placement of the chest (precordial) electrodes

As with the limb electrodes, note any variation from the standard locations on the ECG recording to avoid misinterpretation.

The simplest way to count the rib spaces is to begin by finding the angle of Louis, the horizontal bony ridge part way down the sternum. Run a finger down from the top of the sternum until you feel this ridge, and then run your finger sideways and slightly downwards to the patient's right until you reach a space between the ribs and the right-hand edge of the sternum – the is the second intercostal space. Count down the rib spaces with your fingers to the third and then the fourth intercostal space; this is where you place electrode V1. The equivalent space at the left sternal edge is the location for electrode V2.

Next, staying to the left of the sternum count down to the fifth intercostal space and find the mid-clavicular line – this is the location for electrode V4. Electrode V3 can then be positioned midway between V2 and V4.

Then, move horizontally from electrode V4 to the patient's left until you reach the anterior axillary line. This is the location for electrode V5. It is important to ensure that you do not follow the rib space round to V5, but stay horizontal. Finally, remaining in a horizontal line with V4, place electrode V6 in the mid-axillary line.

FEMALE PATIENTS

Placement of the chest electrodes can sometimes pose difficulties in female patients because of the left breast. By convention, electrodes V4–V6 are placed underneath the left breast.

Special electrode positions

Sometimes it can be helpful to use special positions for the chest electrodes. This is done by moving the usual electrodes to a different location as described in the examples that follow. If this is done, it is essential to label the ECG clearly according to where the electrodes have been placed, as the person interpreting the ECG would not otherwise know that a different position had been used.

Posterior chest leads

Posterior chest leads are useful in identifying a true posterior myocardial infarction (see Chapter 11). To record posterior leads, take three of the chest electrodes (it does not matter which ones) and position them on the posterior aspect of the patient's chest, as shown in Figure 3.3, in the same horizontal plane as V6. These three posterior electrodes are called V7, V8 and V9:

- V7 is placed in the left posterior axillary line.
- V8 is placed at the tip of the left scapula.
- V9 is placed in the left paraspinal region.

When you record the ECG, make sure you annotate the tracing so that it highlights that posterior electrodes have been used, with the V7, V8 and V9 leads clearly labelled and identified.

Right-sided chest leads

Right-sided chest leads are useful in dextrocardia and for identifying right ventricular involvement in an inferior

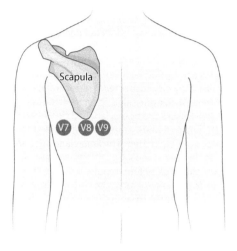

Figure 3.3 Placement of the electrodes to record posterior chest leads. Posterior electrode V8 is placed at the tip of the left scapula, with V7 and V9 placed on either side.

ST segment elevation myocardial infarction (see 'Left ventricular aneurysm' section in Chapter 11). The chest electrodes are placed in a mirror image of their usual positions (Figure 3.4). The chest leads recorded using these electrode positions are conventionally called V1R–V6R, and the ECG must be clearly labelled to show that these electrode positions have been used.

ECG RECORDINGS IN DEXTROCARDIA

In dextrocardia, the heart is located on the right side of the chest rather than on the left. Dextrocardia is suggested by poor R wave progression across the chest leads and by P wave inversion in lead I. If a patient has known or suspected dextrocardia, repeat the recording with right-sided chest electrodes (Figure 3.4). Ensure the ECG is labelled clearly with V1R, V2R, etc. to demonstrate that right-sided chest electrodes have been used. The limb electrodes are usually left in their standard positions, as this helps to 'flag up' the apparent dextrocardia on the ECG, but if you do prefer to reverse the limb electrodes too then it is essential to label the reversed limb leads clearly on the ECG. Ensure that copies of *both* ECGs (the standard one and the one with right-sided electrodes) are retained.

Recording the 12-lead ECG

Enter the patient's name and other relevant identification details (e.g. date of birth, hospital or NHS number) into the ECG machine, and check that the machine is displaying the correct date and time. Many centres now integrate ECG archiving into an electronic patient record, so it's important to ensure that the patient's identification details are correctly recorded digitally.

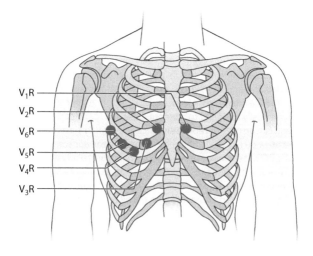

V₁R

V₂R

V₆R

V₅R

V₄R

V₃R

Figure 3.4 Placement of the electrodes to record right-sided chest leads. This is a mirror-image of the standard chest electrode positions.

Encourage the patient to relax while the recording is being made, and check that the patient is lying still and not clenching their muscles.

Do not use a filter for the initial recording; however, if necessary, the recording can be repeated with the filter switched on if the initial recording shows 'noise'.

ECG MACHINE FILTERS

ECG machines offer several types of filters to help improve the quality of the ECG signal. A low-frequency filter is used to filter out low-frequency signals, typically anything less than 0.05 Hz, to reduce baseline drift. A high-frequency filter is used to filter out high-frequency signals, typically anything over 100 Hz, to reduce interference from skeletal muscle. A 'notch' filter is specifically designed to filter out noise at a specific frequency and can be used to reduce electrical alternating current 'hum' at 50 or 60 Hz. While filtering can improve the appearance of the ECG, it can also introduce distortion, particularly of the ST segments, and thus should only be used when necessary. For this reason, ECGs should always initially be recorded with the filters off, and repeated with the filters on only if needed.

ECGs are usually recorded at standard speed and calibration settings. These can be changed by the operator, so always ensure that appropriate settings are used (someone else may have changed the settings on the machine when it was last used).

The standard recording settings are

- Paper speed 25 mm/s
- Gain setting 10 mm/mV

Sometimes these standard settings need to be altered. For example, if an ECG contains high-voltage complexes (as in left ventricular hypertrophy—see Chapter 10), it can be helpful to repeat the recording at a gain setting of 5 mm/mV to reduce the size of the QRS complexes, making the rest of the ECG easier to see. If you make any changes to the settings, ensure that this is clearly marked on the ECG (Figure 3.5). Also,

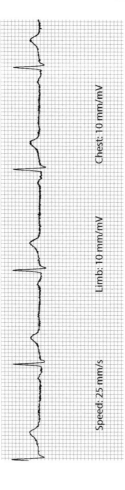

igure 3.5 Paper speed and gain settings as shown on an ECG.

Speed: 25 mm/s   Limb: 10 mm/mV   Chest: 10 mm/mV

be sure to return the machine to its standard settings before you switch it off.

After making the recording

Once the recording has been made, check that it is of good quality and ensure that all the patient details are correctly shown on it.

If the patient was experiencing any symptoms at the time of the recording (such as chest pain or palpitations), note this on the recording as such information can prove very useful diagnostically. Also, if the patient was experiencing symptoms during the recording, or if the recording shows any clinically urgent abnormalities, report this information to a more senior staff member as appropriate.

Once you are satisfied with the ECG recording, detach the electrodes from the patient and assist them in getting dressed. Dispose of any materials used during the recording, such a razors or alcohol wipes, safely and appropriately.

Further reading

Macfarlane PW, Coleman EN. 1995. Resting 12 lead ECG electrode placement and associated problems. Available at www.scst.org.uk, accessed 4 August 2015.

Rudiger A, Hellermann JP, Mukherjee R et al. Electrocardiographic artifacts due to electrode misplacement and their frequency in different clinical settings. *Am J Emerg Med* 2007; **25**: 174–178.

The Society for Cardiological Science and Technology.
2014. Clinical Guidelines by Consensus. Recording
a standard 12-lead electrocardiogram: An approved
methodology by the SCST. Available at www.scst.org.uk,
accessed 4 August 2015.

Chapter 4

How to read a 12-lead ECG

When you read an ECG recording, it's important to do so in a methodical manner to ensure that you don't overlook any potentially important details. In this chapter, we give you a systematic overview of how to read a 12-lead ECG, and in subsequent chapters, we cover many of the individual aspects in more detail.

Patient data

Always begin by checking key information on the ECG and/or request form relating to the patient:

- Patient name
- Patient gender
- Date of birth
- Identification number (e.g. hospital or NHS number)

This will ensure that the ECG relates to the correct individual and also that you take into account any gender- or age-related factors. For instance, the normal values for QTc interval differ for men and women (Chapter 13).

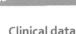

Clinical data

Next, check information on the request form to ascertain
- Reason for the request
- Relevant past medical history
- Relevant medication

This allows you to place your ECG findings in an appropriate clinical context. For instance, is a patient's ST segment depression (Chapter 11) likely to relate to ischaemic heart disease or to treatment with digoxin?

Technical data

Next, review the technical data pertaining to the recording:
- Date and time of recording
- Paper speed and calibration
- Technical quality
- Any unusual aspects to the recording
  - Additional leads (e.g. posterior leads, right-sided chest leads)
  - Diagnostic or therapeutic manoeuvres (e.g. ECG recorded during carotid sinus massage)

Although ECGs are usually recorded at standard settings (see 'Recording the 12-lead ECG' section in Chapter 3), these are sometimes changed (deliberately or accidentally), and this can have a big impact upon subsequent interpretation.

The presence of any technical artefacts, such as electrical interference, also needs to be noted (and ideally the ECG should be repeated, avoiding the artefacts if possible).

ECG fundamentals

Next, review the fundamental features of the ECG recording itself:
- Rate
- Rhythm
  - Supraventricular
  - Ventricular
  - Conduction problems
- Axis

These are the 'traditional' features that begin any ECG interpretation, followed by a more detailed description of the individual features of the recording. You can read more about rate in Chapter 5, rhythm in Chapters 6 through 9 and axis in Chapter 2.

ECG details

Next, review the individual features of the ECG using a step-by-step approach. Describe
- P wave
- PR interval
- Q wave
- QRS complex
- ST segment
- T wave
- QT interval
- U wave

Don't overlook any additional features, such as
- Delta wave (see Figure 7.11)

These features, and how to make sense of any abnormalities, are all discussed in the rest of this book.

Clinical summary

Finally, you need to pull together all your ECG findings and draw a conclusion about what the ECG shows, placing your findings in the context of the clinical information provided. This is where you apply your knowledge of the ECG, and what each ECG feature can indicate, in order to draw conclusions about the patient's condition.

You may need to describe your ECG findings to another healthcare professional, or to document your findings in the patient's casenotes. A comprehensive ECG report may read like this:

This 12-lead ECG was performed on John Smith, born on 1 January 1950, hospital number 123456. The request form states that the patient is experiencing breathlessness and irregular palpitations. He has a history of inferior myocardial infarction in 2011. He is currently taking aspirin, atorvastatin, bisoprolol and ramipril.

The recording was performed on 1 August 2015, using a paper speed of 25 mm/s and a calibration of 10 mm/mV. The recording is of good quality with no artefact.

The ventricular rate is tachycardic at 114 beats/min. The rhythm is atrial fibrillation, as evidenced by no coordinated atrial activity and irregularly irregular QRS complexes. The QRS axis is normal at +64°.

The P waves are absent and so the PR interval cannot be measured. There are deep Q waves and inverted T waves in the inferior leads. The remainder of the QRS complexes are unremarkable. The ST segments are normal. The QT interval is normal (QT_c measures 428 ms). There are no U waves present.

In conclusion, this 12-lead ECG shows:

- Atrial fibrillation with a fast ventricular rate (114 beats/min)
- Inferior Q waves and T wave inversion, consistent with an old inferior myocardial infarction

If you have old ECGs for comparison, you may wish to include details of any relevant changes in the ECG as well (e.g. new evidence of myocardial infarction and new conduction problems, changes in rhythm).

Further reading

Mason JW, Hancock EW, Gettes LS. AHA/ACCF/HRS recommendations for the standardization and interpretation of the electrocardiogram: Part II: Electrocardiography diagnostic statement list. *J Am Coll Cardiol* 2007; **49**: 1128–1135.

Chapter 5

Heart rate: Bradycardia and tachycardia

Calculating heart rate is fundamental to ECG interpretation, as it is a key step in the recognition of arrhythmias. In the next few chapters, we will be looking at heart rhythms in detail, but let us begin by describing ways to measure heart rate and the abnormalities that can affect it.

The term 'heart rate' usually means the *ventricular* rate, which corresponds to the patient's pulse. Depolarization of the ventricles produces the QRS complex on the ECG, and so it is the rate of QRS complexes that needs to be measured to determine heart rate.

The measurement of heart rate is simple and can be done in several ways. However, before you try to measure anything, check that the ECG has been recorded at the standard paper speed of 25 mm/s. All the methods described in this chapter apply to ECGs performed at the standard paper speed.

Method 1: Counting large squares

ECG recording paper has a standard grid of large and small squares pre-printed on it. Each large square is 5 mm wide. If the ECG has been recorded at a paper speed of 25 mm/s, then a 1 min ECG tracing covers *300 large squares* on the ECG paper.

If the patient's ventricular rhythm is regular, then all the QRS complexes will be the same distance apart, and all you have to do is count the number of large squares between two consecutive QRS complexes and divide it into 300. For example, in Figure 5.1, there are approximately four large squares between each QRS complex. Therefore:

$$\text{Heart rate} = \frac{300}{4} = 75 \text{ beats/min}$$

This method will give you an approximate heart rate, but only works when the rhythm is regular. If the rhythm is irregular, then the number of large squares will vary between one QRS complex and the next.

Method 2: Counting small squares

An alternative, and slightly more accurate, method is to count small squares rather than big ones. Each small square is 1 mm wide. If the ECG has been recorded at a paper speed of 25 mm/s, then a 1 min ECG tracing covers *1500 small squares* on the ECG paper.

Count the number of small squares between two consecutive

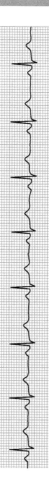

Figure 5.1 Calculating heart rate when the rhythm is regular. There are approximately four large squares between each QRS complex, corresponding to a heart rate of approximately 75 beats/min. More precisely, there are 21 small squares between each QRS complex, giving a more accurate heart rate of 71 beats/min.

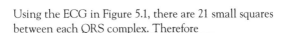

Using the ECG in Figure 5.1, there are 21 small squares between each QRS complex. Therefore

$$\text{Heart rate} = \frac{1500}{21} = 71 \text{ beats/min}$$

This is similar to the result of 75 beats/min that we got by counting the big squares, but is slightly more accurate. Like the big square method, the small square method does not work when the rhythm is irregular. In this case, we should use method 3.

Method 3: Counting QRS complexes

When the patient's heart rhythm is irregular, the number of large and small squares between each QRS complex varies from beat to beat. A more effective method for calculating ventricular rate in this situation is to simply count the number of QRS complexes in 50 large squares (Figure 5.2) – the length of the rhythm strip on standard ECG.

At a standard paper speed of 25 mm/s, a rhythm strip measuring 50 large squares equates to 10 s in time. Therefore if you count up the number of QRS complexes in 50 large squares, this is the same as the number of QRS complexes occurring over a period of 10 s. To convert this to a rate in beats/min, simply multiply by 6:

Number of QRS complexes in 50 large squares = 19

Therefore, number of QRS complexes in 10 s = 19

Therefore, number of QRS complexes/min = 19 × 6 = 114

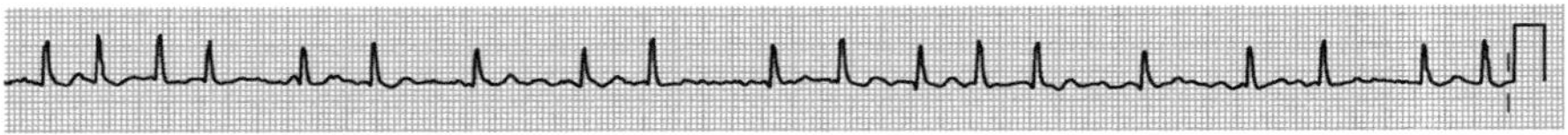

Figure 5.2 Calculating heart rate when the rhythm is irregular. There are 19 QRS complexes in 50 large squares (10 s), corresponding to a heart rate of 114 beats/min.

This method of counting the QRS complexes works regardless of whether the rhythm is irregular or regular.

AUTOMATED HEART RATE CALCULATIONS

Some ECG machines will calculate heart rate automatically and print it on the ECG, but always check machine-derived values, as the machines do occasionally make errors!

P wave rate

Whichever method you use for calculating ventricular (QRS complex) rate, remember it can also be used to measure the atrial (P wave) rate.

Normally, every P wave is followed by a QRS complex and so the atrial and ventricular rates are the same. However, the P wave and QRS complex rates can be different if, for example, some or all of the P waves are prevented from activating the ventricles, as seen in third-degree atrioventricular (AV) block (Figure 5.3). Situations where this may happen are described in Chapter 9.

Bradycardia and tachycardia

Once you have measured the heart rate, you need to decide whether it is normal or abnormal. A ventricular rate between 60 and 100 beats/min is regarded as normal. If the rate is below 60 beats/min, the patient is said to be *bradycardic*. With a heart rate above 100 beats/min, the

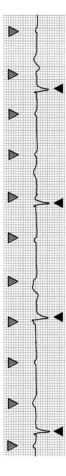

Figure 5.3 The P wave rate can differ from the QRS complex rate. This rhythm strip shows third-degree AV block, with the P waves indicated by red arrowheads and the QRS complexes by black arrowheads. The P wave (atrial) rate is 94/min versus a QRS complex (ventricular) rate of 33 beats/min.

Causes of bradycardia

Bradycardia is defined as a heart rate below 60 beats/min (Figure 5.4). There can be many causes for this, and in Chapters 6 through 9, we will look in detail at the range of heart rhythms and conduction problems that can be responsible for a patient becoming bradycardic. Common problems to consider in a bradycardic patient are

- Sinus bradycardia
- Sick sinus syndrome
- Second-degree and third-degree AV block
- 'Escape' rhythms
  - AV junctional escape rhythm
  - Ventricular escape rhythms
- Asystole

Sinus bradycardia (see Chapter 7) can be normal (in athletes, or during sleep). The differential diagnosis and treatment are discussed in Chapter 7.

Sick sinus syndrome (see Chapter 7) is the coexistence of sinus bradycardia with episodes of sinus arrest and sinoatrial block. Patients may also have episodes of paroxysmal tachycardia, giving rise to the tachy-brady syndrome.

In *second-degree AV block* (see Chapter 9) some atrial impulses fail to be conducted to the ventricles, and this can lead to bradycardia. In *third-degree AV block*, no atrial impulses can reach the ventricles; in response, the ventricles usually develop an 'escape' rhythm (see next). It is important to remember that AV block can coexist with *any* atrial rhythm.

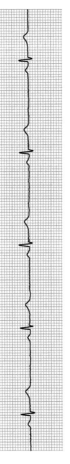

Figure 5.4 Sinus bradycardia. Heart rate is 46 beats/min.

Escape rhythms are a form of 'safety net' to maintain a heart beat if the normal mechanism of impulse generation fails or is blocked. They may also appear during episodes of severe sinus bradycardia. Escape rhythms are discussed in more detail in Chapter 9.

Asystole (see 'Is ventricular activity present?' section in Chapter 6) implies the absence of ventricular activity, and so the heart rate is zero. Asystole is a medical emergency and requires immediate diagnosis and treatment if the patient is to have any chance of survival.

BRADYCARDIA CAUSED BY DRUG TREATMENT

Certain drugs can slow heart rate and cause a bradycardia. These are known as *negatively chronotropic* drugs. This can occur even if the patient's original heart rate was normal or fast – for example patients with atrial fibrillation (which if untreated often causes a *tachycardia*) can develop a *bradycardia* when commenced on anti-arrhythmic drugs. Table 5.1 lists drugs that commonly slow heart rate. Always review current and recent medication if a patient is bradycardic.

Table 5.1 Common negatively chronotropic drugs

• Beta blockers (do not forget eye drops)
• Some calcium antagonists, for example verapamil, diltiazem
• Digoxin
• Ivabradine

The first step in managing a bradycardia is to assess the urgency of the situation – in the peri-arrest situation, use the ABCDE approach and assess the patient for adverse features (see 'Is ventricular activity present?' section in Chapter 6). The Resuscitation Council (UK) 2015 algorithm on the immediate management of bradycardia in adults is shown in Figure 5.5.

Causes of tachycardia

Tachycardia is defined as a heart rate above 100 beats/min (Figure 5.6). As with bradycardia, there can be many causes for this, and in Chapters 6 through 9, we will consider these in detail. Tachycardias can be considered in two groups, depending upon the width of the QRS complexes. To start the process of identifying a tachycardia, check whether the QRS complexes are

- Narrow (<3 small squares)
- Broad (>3 small squares)

Narrow-complex tachycardias always arise from *above* the ventricles – that is to say, they are *supraventricular* in origin. The possibilities are

- Sinus tachycardia
- Atrial tachycardia
- Atrial flutter
- Atrial fibrillation
- AV re-entry tachycardia (AVRT)
- AV nodal re-entry tachycardia (AVNRT)

All of these are discussed in Chapter 7.

Broad QRS complexes can occur if normal electrical impulses are conducted abnormally ('aberrantly') to

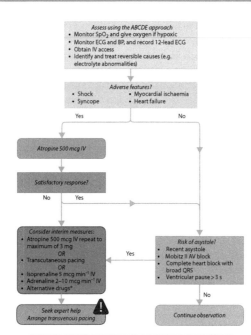

Figure 5.5 Resuscitation Council (UK) 2015 adult bradycardia algorithm. ABCDE, Airway, Breathing, Circulation, Disability, Exposure (see 'How is the patient?' section in Chapter 6); BP, blood pressure; IV, intravenous. (Reproduced with the kind permission of the Resuscitation Council, London, UK, *Resuscitation Guidelines 2015*, https://www.resus.org.uk/resuscitation-guidelines/peri-

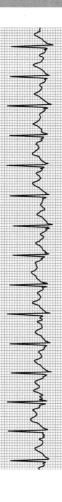

Figure 5.6 Sinus tachycardia. Heart rate is 136 beats/min.

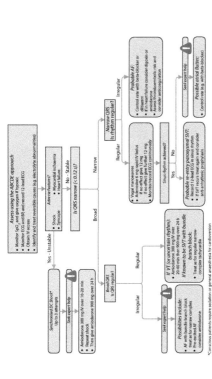

Figure 5.7 Resuscitation Council (UK) 2015 adult tachycardia (with a pulse) algorithm. ABCDE, Airway, Breathing, Circulation, Disability, Exposure (see 'How is the patient?' section in Chapter 6); AF, atrial fibrillation; BP, blood pressure; IV, intravenous; SVT, supraventricular tachycardia; VT, ventricular tachycardia. (Reproduced with the kind permission of the Resuscitation Council, London, UK, *Resuscitation Guidelines 2015*, https://www.resus.org.uk/resuscitation-guidelines/peri-arrest-arrhythmias/, accessed 18 October 2015.)

the ventricles. This delays ventricular activation, widening the QRS complex. Any of the supraventricular tachycardias (SVTs) listed here can also present as a *broad-complex tachycardia* if aberrant conduction is present. Broad-complex tachycardia should also make you think of ventricular arrhythmias:

- Ventricular tachycardia
- Accelerated idioventricular rhythm
- Torsades de pointes

Each of these is discussed in Chapter 8. A common question that arises with broad-complex tachycardia is how to tell the difference between ventricular tachycardia and SVT with aberrant conduction. This is discussed in the 'Is this VT or SVT with aberrant conduction?' section in Chapter 8.

Ventricular fibrillation (VF, see Chapter 8) is hard to categorize. The chaotic nature of the underlying ventricular activity can give rise to a variety of ECG appearances, but all have the characteristics of being unpredictable and chaotic. Ventricular fibrillation is a cardiac arrest rhythm and so it is essential that you can recognize it immediately.

Management of tachycardia depends on the underlying rhythm. The first step, as with managing a bradycardia, is to assess the urgency of the situation – in the peri-arrest situation, use the ABCDE approach and assess the patient for adverse features. The Resuscitation Council (UK) 2015 algorithm on the immediate management of tachycardia (with a pulse) in adults is shown in Figure 5.7.

Further reading

Details of Advanced Life Support guidelines, and training courses in resuscitation, can be obtained from the Resuscitation Council, London, UK. At: http://www.resus.org.uk/, accessed 4 August 2015.

Meek S, Morri F. ABC of clinical electrocardiography: Introduction. I – Leads, rate, rhythm, and cardiac axis. *Br Med J* 2002; **324**: 415–418.

Chapter 6

An approach to heart rhythms

Just as you need to have a systematic approach to the 12-lead ECG, it also helps if you take a structured approach to identifying heart rhythms. In the last chapter, we considered abnormalities of heart rate – bradycardia and tachycardia. In this chapter, we'll take a step-by-step approach to the recognition of normal and abnormal heart rhythms.

To identify the cardiac rhythm with confidence, you need to begin with a *rhythm strip* – a prolonged recording of the ECG. Most ECG machines automatically include a rhythm strip at the bottom of a 12-lead ECG (Figure 6.1). If your machine does not, make sure you have recorded one yourself. The machine may give you a choice about which of the 12 leads will appear as the rhythm strip – most commonly, lead II is selected as this tends to give the clearest view of the P wave activity.

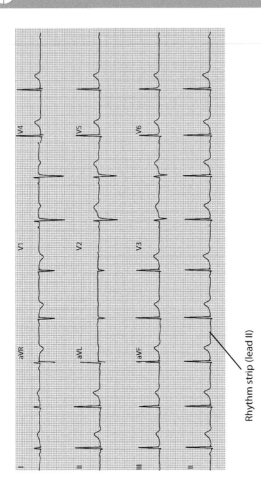

Rhythm strip (lead II)

Figure 6.1 The rhythm strip. The standard lead used for the rhythm strip is lead II, but alternative leads can be selected if it helps to clarify the cardiac rhythm.

Identifying the cardiac rhythm

There are many ways in which you can approach the identification of arrhythmias, and this is reflected in the numerous ways in which they can be categorized:

- Regular versus irregular
- Bradycardias versus tachycardias
- Narrow complex versus broad complex
- Supraventricular versus ventricular.

When you analyse the cardiac rhythm, always keep in mind the two primary questions that you are trying to answer:

1. Where does the impulse arise from?
   - Sinoatrial (SA) node
   - Atria
   - Atrioventricular (AV) junction
   - Ventricles
2. How is the impulse conducted?
   - Normal conduction
   - Impaired conduction
   - Accelerated conduction (e.g. Wolff–Parkinson–White syndrome).

We will help you to narrow down the possibilities with the following seven questions:

1. How is the patient?
2. Is ventricular activity present?
3. What is the ventricular rate?
4. Is the ventricular rhythm regular or irregular?
5. Is the QRS complex width normal or broad?
6. Is atrial activity present?
7. How are atrial activity and ventricular activity related?

How is the patient?

Clinical context is all important in ECG interpretation, and so don't attempt to interpret an ECG rhythm without knowing the clinical context in which the ECG was recorded. For instance, the presence of artefact on an ECG can be misread as an arrhythmia unless the clinical context is known. Do the following to avoid these problems:

- If you are interpreting an ECG that someone else has recorded, always ask for the clinical details of the patient and the reason why it was recorded.
- If you are recording an ECG that someone else will interpret later, always make a note of relevant clinical details at the top of the ECG to help with the interpretation (e.g. 'Patient experiencing chest pain at time of recording').

The clinical context will also help you decide how urgently to deal with an arrhythmia. When assessing a 'sick' patient, use the *ABCDE* approach:

- *Airway* – Check for any evidence of airway obstruction.
- *Breathing* – Assess the patient's breathing, paying attention to respiratory rate, chest examination and oxygenation.
- *Circulation* – Assess the patient's circulation, including pulse rate, blood pressure and capillary refill time.
- *Disability* – Assess the level of consciousness and neurological status.
- *Exposure/examination* – Ensure adequate exposure to permit a full examination.

As you assess a patient with an arrhythmia, be alert for so-called 'adverse features' which indicate haemodynamic instability:

- *Shock* – As evidenced by hypotension (systolic blood pressure <90 mmHg), clamminess, sweating, pallor, confusion or reduced conscious level.
- *Syncope* – As a consequence of cerebral hypoperfusion.
- *Myocardial ischaemia* – Indicated by ischaemic chest pain and/or ischaemic ECG changes (Chapter 11).
- *Heart failure* – Pulmonary oedema, elevated jugular venous pressure, peripheral/sacral oedema.

Once you've established the clinical context of the ECG recording, move on to the next question.

Is ventricular activity present?

Examine the ECG as a whole for the presence of QRS complexes (which indicate ventricular electrical activity). If no QRS complexes are present, check

- The patient (Do they have a pulse?)
- The electrodes (Has something become disconnected?)
- The gain setting (Is the gain setting on the monitor too low?)

If the patient is pulseless with no electrical activity evident on the ECG, they are in *asystole* and appropriate emergency action must be taken – see Figure 8.6 for more details. Beware of diagnosing asystole in the presence of a *completely* flat ECG trace – there should usually be some baseline 'drift' present (Figure 6.2). A completely flat line usually means an electrode has become disconnected – check the electrodes (and, of course, the patient) carefully when making your diagnosis.

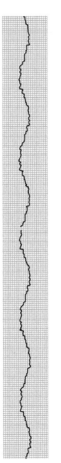

Figure 6.2 Asystole. There is no evidence of ventricular electrical activity (complete absence of QRS complexes). Note the presence of baseline 'drift'.

P waves may appear on their own (for a short time) after the onset of ventricular asystole. The presence of 'P waves only' on the ECG is important to recognize, as the patient may respond to emergency pacing manoeuvres such as temporary pacing.

If QRS complexes are present, move on to the next question.

What is the ventricular rate?

Ventricular activity is represented on the ECG by QRS complexes. Three methods for determining the ventricular rate have already been discussed in Chapter 5. Once you have calculated the ventricular rate, you will be able to classify the rhythm as:

- Bradycardia (<60 beats/min)
- Normal (60–100 beats/min)
- Tachycardia (>100 beats/min).

Having calculated the ventricular rate, move on to the next question.

Is the ventricular rhythm regular or irregular?

To assess the regularity of the ventricular rhythm, look carefully at the spacing between the QRS complexes – is it the same throughout the rhythm strip? Irregularity can be subtle, so it is useful to measure out the distance between each QRS complex. One way to do this is to place a piece of paper alongside the rhythm strip and make a mark on it next to every QRS complex. By moving the marked paper up and down along the rhythm strip, you can soon see if the gaps between the QRS complexes are the same or vary.

Once you have assessed the regularity, you will be able to classify the ventricular rhythm as

- Regular (equal spacing between QRS complexes)
- Irregular (variable spacing between QRS complexes)

Table 6.1 lists the causes of regular and irregular cardiac rhythms.

Once you have determined whether the rhythm is regular or irregular, move on to the next question.

'REGULAR' VERSUS 'IRREGULAR' IRREGULARITY

You may encounter the terms 'regularly irregular' and 'irregularly irregular' used in relation to irregular rhythm. This is because some rhythms can be chaotic (e.g. atrial fibrillation, Figure 7.6) where it is impossible to predict where the next QRS complex will occur: this is called 'irregularly irregular'. However, some irregular rhythms are predictable – there may be an 'extra' beat (e.g. bigeminy, Figure 8.2) or a 'missing' beat (e.g. Mobitz type 1 AV block, Figure 9.3) that occurs in a regular pattern, so although the overall rhythm is irregular, the irregularity is predictable. This is a 'regularly irregular' rhythm.

Is the QRS complex width normal or broad?

The width of the QRS complex can provide valuable clues about where the cardiac rhythm has originated. By answering this question, you may therefore be able to narrow down the origin of the rhythm to one half of

Table 6.1 Regular and irregular cardiac rhythms

• Regular rhythms
• Sinus rhythm
• Sinus bradycardia
• Sinus tachycardia
• Atrial flutter (if constant AV block, e.g. 2:1)
• Atrial tachycardia
– AV re-entry tachycardia (AVRT)
– AV nodal re-entry tachycardia (AVNRT)
• Accelerated idioventricular rhythm
• Monomorphic ventricular tachycardia (VT)
• Polymorphic ventricular tachycardia ('torsades de pointes')
• Second-degree AV block
– 2:1 AV block
• Third-degree AV block (if regular escape rhythm)
• Irregular rhythms
• Sinus arrhythmia (rate varies with respiration)
• Ectopic beats (atrial, junctional, ventricular)
• Atrial fibrillation
• Atrial flutter (if there is variable AV block)
• Sinus arrest and SA block
• Second-degree AV block
– Mobitz type 1 AV block
– Mobitz type 2 AV block

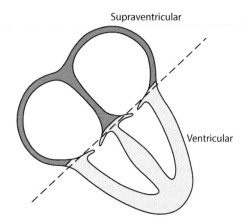

Figure 6.3 Supraventricular versus ventricular rhythms.
Supraventricular applies to any structure above the ventricles
(and electrically distinct from them).

ventricular myocardium; supraventricular rhythms are
generated anywhere up to (and including) the AV junction
(Figure 6.3).

As we learned in Chapter 1, the ventricles are normally
depolarized via the His–Purkinje system, a network
of rapidly conducting fibres that runs throughout the
ventricular myocardium. As a result, the ventricles are
normally completely depolarized within 0.12 s, and that is
why the QRS complex on the ECG is narrow (less than
three small squares wide).

However, if there is a problem with conduction within the

(as seen in left or right bundle branch block), the ventricles can no longer make full use of this rapid conduction system to depolarize. Instead, in areas of the heart where this rapid conduction system is blocked, depolarization has to travel slowly from myocyte to myocyte instead. This takes longer, and so the QRS complex becomes *broader* than three small squares. This is also the case if the impulse has arisen within the ventricles (instead of coming via the AV node), as in the case of a ventricular ectopic beat or in ventricular tachycardia (VT). If an impulse does not pass through the AV node, it cannot make use of the His–Purkinje conduction system (as the only way to get into this system is via the AV node). Once again, the impulse is obliged to travel slowly from myocyte to myocyte, prolonging the process of depolarization.

This explains why the QRS complexes are broad when there is a left or right bundle branch block. It also explains why ventricular ectopics are broad, and why VT is a broad-complex tachycardia.

So we can now use this information to try to determine how the ventricles were depolarized. If the QRS complex is narrow (<3 small squares), the ventricles must have been rapidly depolarized by an impulse that came through the AV node – the only way into the His–Purkinje system. The patient is then said to have a *supraventricular rhythm* (arising from above the ventricles).

If the QRS complex is broad (>3 small squares), there are two possible explanations:

1. The impulse may have arisen from within the ventricles and thus been unable to travel via the His–Purkinje

Table 6.2 Broad-complex versus narrow-complex rhythms

Rhythm origin	Rhythm conduction	QRS complex
Supraventricular	Normal	Narrow
Supraventricular	Aberrant (e.g. bundle branch block)	Broad
Ventricular	Myocyte-to-myocyte	Broad

Note: Only supraventricular rhythms with normal conduction can gain access to the His–Purkinje system and depolarize the ventricles rapidly.

2. The impulse may have arisen from above the ventricles but not been able to use all the His–Purkinje system because of a conduction problem (*supraventricular rhythm with aberrant conduction*).

This is summarized in Table 6.2.

Once you have assessed whether the QRS complexes are narrow or broad, move on to the next question.

Is atrial activity present?

Atrial electrical activity can take several forms, which can be grouped into four categories:

1. P waves (atrial depolarization)
2. Flutter waves (atrial flutter)
3. Fibrillation waves (atrial fibrillation)
4. Unclear activity

The presence of *P waves* indicates atrial depolarization. This does not mean that the depolarization necessarily started at the SA node, however. P waves will appear during atrial depolarization regardless of where it originated – it is the *orientation* of the P waves that tells you where the depolarization originated. Upright P waves in lead II suggest that atrial depolarization originated in or near the SA node. Inverted P waves suggest an origin closer to, or within, the AV node (Figure 7.9).

Flutter waves are seen in atrial flutter at a rate of 300/min, creating a sawtooth baseline of atrial activity (Figure 7.7). This can be made more readily apparent by manoeuvres that transiently block the AV node (page 7.8).

Fibrillation waves are seen in AF and correspond to random, chaotic atrial impulses occurring at a rate of around 400–600/min (Figure 7.6). This leads to a chaotic, low-amplitude baseline of atrial activity.

The nature of the atrial activity may be *unclear*. This may be because P waves are 'hidden' within the QRS complexes, as is often the case during AV nodal re-entry tachycardia. In such cases, atrial depolarization *is* taking place, but its electrical 'signature' on the ECG cannot easily be seen because the simultaneous, larger amplitude, QRS complex hides it. Atrial activity may also be absent in, for example, sinus arrest or SA block, in which case the atria may be electrically silent.

Once you have assessed whether atrial activity is present, move on to the final question.

How are atrial activity and ventricular activity related?

In the previous six steps, you have examined the activity of the atria and of the ventricles. The final task is to determine how the two are related.

In normal sinus rhythm, with no conduction problems, every

leading to a 1:1 relationship between P waves and QRS complexes. However, in some conditions, impulses from the atria may fail to reach the ventricles, or the ventricles may generate their own impulses independent of the atria.

Take a careful look at the P waves and the QRS complexes, and assess whether the two are related. If every QRS complex is associated with a P wave, this indicates that the atria and ventricles are being activated by a common source. This is usually, but not necessarily, the SA node (e.g. AV junctional rhythms will also depolarize both atria and ventricles).

However, if there are more P waves than QRS complexes, conduction between atria and ventricles is being either partly blocked (with only some impulses getting through) or completely blocked (with the ventricles having developed their own escape rhythm). Conduction problems are discussed further in Chapter 9.

If there are more QRS complexes than P waves, this indicates AV dissociation (see 'Is this VT or SVT with aberrant conduction?' section in Chapter 8), with the ventricles operating independently of the atria and at a higher rate.

Determining the cardiac rhythm

The seven steps discussed will give you a systematic method for approaching ECG rhythms. As you read about supraventricular rhythms, ventricular rhythms and conduction problems in the next three chapters, think about these seven questions and how they relate to each of the rhythms described. Each rhythm has its own set of ECG characteristics, and by assessing the

ECG in a systematic manner you will quickly learn how to distinguish between them.

> **IF IN DOUBT...**
>
> The recognition of arrhythmias can be tricky, and making the correct diagnosis can have significant implications for how a patient is treated. Some of the more complex arrhythmias can tax the skills of even the most senior members of the cardiology team. If in doubt about a patient's cardiac rhythm, do not hesitate to seek the advice of an experienced colleague.

Further reading

Wellens HJJ. Ventricular tachycardia: Diagnosis of broad QRS complex tachycardia. *Heart* 2001; **86**: 579–585.

Whinnett ZI, Sohaib SMA, Davies DW. Diagnosis and management of supraventricular tachycardia. *BMJ* 2012; **345**: e7769.

Chapter 7

Supraventricular rhythms

Supraventricular rhythms are those which originate above the level of the ventricles, that is from the sinoatrial (SA) node, the atria or the atrioventricular (AV) node (Figure 6.3). There are several different supraventricular rhythms and all of these are discussed in this chapter.

Sinus rhythm

Sinus rhythm is the normal cardiac rhythm, in which the SA node acts as the natural pacemaker, discharging at a rate of 60–100 beats/min (Figure 7.1). In sinus rhythm, every P wave is followed by a QRS complex, and the P wave morphology is normal (e.g. upright in lead II and inverted in lead aVR).

Sinus arrhythmia

Sinus arrhythmia describes the *normal* variation in heart rate that can be seen during inspiration and expiration (Figure 7.2). This is sinus rhythm, but with a physiological

ead II

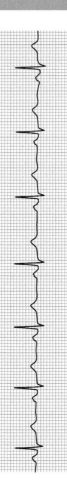

igure 7.1 Normal sinus rhythm. The heart rate is 75 beats/min, the P waves are upright (lead II) and very P wave is followed by a QRS complex.

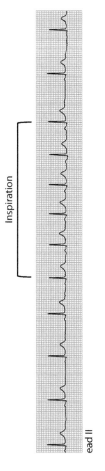

ead II

igure 7.2 Physiological sinus arrhythmia. The heart rate increases during inspiration and decreases uring expiration.

variation in rate due to the blood flow changes that occur with respiration:

- During *inspiration*, the heart rate *increases* as a reflex response to the increased volume of blood returning to the heart
- During *expiration*, the heart rate *decreases* as a reflex response to the decreased volume of blood returning to the heart.

Sinus arrhythmia is harmless and no investigations or treatment are necessary.

Sinus bradycardia

Sinus bradycardia is sinus rhythm with a heart rate of less than 60 beats/min (Figure 7.3). Mild sinus bradycardia (40–60 beats/min) can be normal, for example in athletes or during sleep. However, always consider:

- Negatively chronotropic drugs (Table 5.1)
- Myocardial ischaemia/infarction
- Hypothyroidism
- Hypothermia
- Electrolyte abnormalities
- Raised intracranial pressure
- Sick sinus syndrome

Symptomatic sinus bradycardia is treated by correction of the underlying cause (where appropriate) or, if necessary, consideration of pacing.

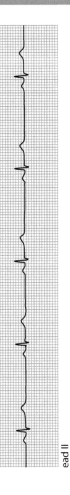

ead II

igure 7.3 Sinus bradycardia. The heart rate is 46 beats/min, the P waves are upright (lead II) and very P wave is followed by a QRS complex.

Sinus tachycardia

Sinus tachycardia is sinus rhythm with a heart rate of greater
than 100 beats/min (Figure 7.4). Physiological causes include
anything that stimulates the sympathetic nervous system –
anxiety, pain, fear, fever or exercise. Also, always consider

- Drugs, e.g. adrenaline, atropine, salbutamol (do not forget
  inhalers and nebulizers), caffeine and alcohol
- Myocardial ischaemia/infarction
- Hyperthyroidism
- Heart failure
- Pulmonary embolism
- Fluid loss
- Anaemia

It is unusual for sinus tachycardia to exceed 180 beats/min,
except in fit athletes. At this heart rate, it may be difficult
to differentiate the P waves from the T waves, so the rhythm
can be mistaken for an AV nodal re-entry tachycardia
(see Chapter 7).

The treatment of sinus tachycardia is usually that of the
underlying cause.

Sick sinus syndrome

As the name suggests, sick sinus syndrome is a collection
of impulse generation and conduction problems related to
dysfunction of the sinus node. Any, or all, of the following
problems may occur:

- Sinus bradycardia
- Sinus tachycardia
- Sinus arrest

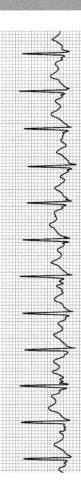

Lead II

Figure 7.4 Sinus tachycardia. The heart rate is 136 beats/min, the P waves are upright (lead II) and every P wave is followed by a QRS complex.

In *sinus arrest*, the sinus node sometimes fails to discharge on time – looking at a rhythm strip, a P wave will suddenly fail to appear in the expected place, and there is a gap, of variable length, until the next P wave appears. In *SA block*, the sinus node depolarizes as normal, but the impulse fails to reach the atria. A P wave fails to appear in the expected place, but the next one usually appears exactly where it is expected.

Sick sinus syndrome may also coexist with tachycardias such as atrial fibrillation (AF), atrial flutter or atrial tachycardia. The association of sick sinus syndrome with paroxysmal tachycardias is called *tachycardia–bradycardia* (or 'tachy-brady') *syndrome*.

Sick sinus syndrome, and the associated tachy-brady syndrome, may cause symptoms of dizziness, fainting and palpitation. Asymptomatic patients do not require treatment. Patients with symptoms need consideration of a permanent pacemaker.

Atrial ectopic beats

Ectopic beats appear *earlier* than expected and are therefore identified by a P wave that appears early and has a different shape to the normal P waves (Figure 7.5). Atrial ectopic beats will usually (but not always) be conducted to the ventricles and therefore be followed by a QRS complex. Atrial ectopic beats are also called atrial extrasystoles, atrial premature complexes (APCs), atrial premature beats (APBs) or premature atrial contractions (PACs). Atrial ectopic beats are a common finding in normal individuals and do not usually need treatment unless they cause troublesome symptoms, in

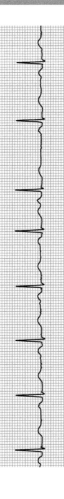

ead II

igure 7.5 Atrial ectopic beat. After five normal sinus beats, the sixth beat is an atrial ectopic. occurs earlier than expected, and the shape of the P wave is different to that of the normal waves in sinus rhythm, indicating an origin in a different part of the atria.

Atrial fibrillation

AF is a common and important arrhythmia, and is associated with an increased risk of stroke. The basis of AF is rapid, chaotic depolarization occurring throughout the atria. No P waves are seen and the ECG baseline consists of low-amplitude oscillations (Figure 7.6).

Although around 400–600 impulses reach the AV node every minute, only some will be transmitted to the ventricles. The ventricular rate is typically fast (100–180 beats/min), although the rate can be normal or even slow. Transmission of the atrial impulses through the AV node is erratic, making the ventricular rhythm 'irregularly irregular'.

AF can be persistent (continuous AF lasting >7 days or requiring cardioversion) or paroxysmal (self-terminating episodes, typically lasting <48 h although they can last up to 7 days). AF may be asymptomatic, but many patients will experience palpitation, breathlessness and/or fatigue.

Reducing stroke risk

AF increases a patient's stroke risk fivefold, and one in five strokes occurs as a result of AF. Reducing stroke risk in AF is therefore important. Stroke risk can be formally assessed using the CHA_2DS_2-VASc scoring system, but in general the approach can be summarized as follows:

- For patients with valvular AF (including rheumatic valve disease and prosthetic valves), anticoagulation with warfarin is recommended for all, unless there are contraindications.

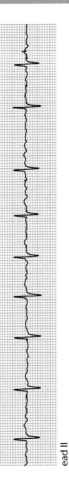

Lead II

Figure 7.6 Atrial fibrillation. The ventricular rhythm is irregularly irregular, with an absence of distinct P waves.

- For those with non-valvular AF, anticoagulation (using warfarin or one of the newer oral anticoagulants, such as dabigatran) is recommended for all, except in those patients who are at low risk (aged <65 years and lone AF), or with contraindications.

Ventricular rate control

Where patients have a rapid ventricular rate, the heart can be slowed using beta blockers or non-dihydropyridine calcium channel blockers (verapamil or diltiazem). Digoxin is good for rate control at rest but is poor at rate control during exercise.

Initially, a 'lenient' rate control strategy can be adopted, aiming for a resting ventricular rate <110 beats/min.

If patients remain symptomatic, a stricter rate control strategy can be used, aiming for a resting heart rate <80 beats/min (with a heart rate <110 beats/min during moderate exercise). If drug therapy cannot attain satisfactory rate control in AF, and restoration of sinus rhythm cannot be achieved, an alternative strategy is to undertake ablation of the AV node plus permanent pacing. This places the patient in complete heart block, and they are then pacemaker-dependent.

Rhythm control

Patients with symptomatic AF despite adequate ventricular rate control should be considered for a rhythm control strategy, where the aim is to restore and maintain sinus rhythm. The can be attempted electrically (DC cardioversion) or pharmacologically ('chemical' chosen according to current guidelines. Another option, particularly for paroxysmal AF, is electrophysiological catheter ablation which usually involves electrical isolation of the pulmonary veins.

Atrial flutter

Atrial flutter is most commonly due to an impulse looping in a circuit around the right atrium. It takes about 0.2 s for the impulse to complete a circuit, each time giving rise to a wave of depolarization and a flutter wave on the ECG. There are thus about five flutter waves every second, and so around 300 every minute (Figure 7.7). The flutter waves give a characteristic 'sawtooth' appearance to the baseline of the ECG.

In atrial flutter the AV node cannot normally keep up with atrial impulses at such a high rate and so AV block occurs. This is commonly 2:1 block, which means that only alternate atrial impulses get through the AV node to initiate a QRS complex. In some cases 3:1, 4:1 or variable degrees of block (Figure 7.8) are also seen. Thus, the ventricular rate is less than the atrial rate, and is often 150, 100, or 75 beats/min. You should therefore always suspect atrial flutter with 2:1 block when a patient has a regular tachycardia with a ventricular rate of about 150 beats/min.

The management of atrial flutter is similar to AF (see 'Atrial fibrillation' section) with anticoagulation, rate control and cardioversion as appropriate. Electrophysiological ablation of the atrial flutter circuit is also an option, with a success

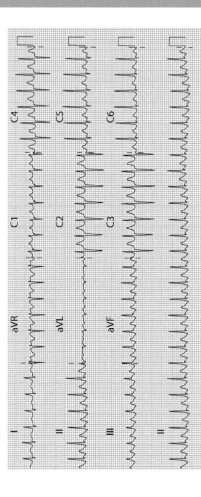

Figure 7.7 Atrial flutter. There is a 'sawtooth' pattern of atrial activity, with an atrial rate of 300 beats/min and a ventricular rate of 150 beats/min (indicating 2:1 AV block).

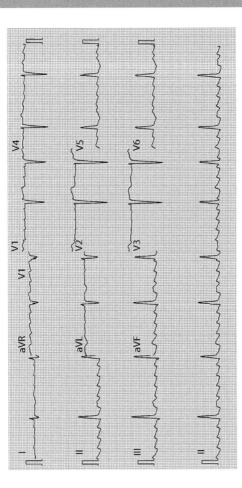

Figure 7.8 Atrial flutter. There is a 'sawtooth' pattern of atrial activity, with an atrial rate of 250 beats/min and a ventricular rate of 48 beats/min. The ventricular rhythm is irregular, indicating variable AV block.

Atrial tachycardia

Atrial tachycardia is an arrhythmia in which the impulses are generated by an ectopic focus somewhere within the atrial myocardium (other than the sinus node). The atrial rate is usually 100–250 beats/min, with abnormally shaped P waves (Figure 7.9). Above atrial rates of 200 beats/min, the AV node struggles to keep up with impulse conduction and AV block may occur.

Brief episodes of atrial tachycardia are commonly seen during ECG monitoring, and are often asymptomatic. Sustained atrial tachycardia can lead to a tachycardia-induced cardiomyopathy, and it is particularly important not to misdiagnose the rhythm as sinus tachycardia in such cases.

Atrial tachycardia can be rate-controlled with beta blockers or non-dihydropyridine calcium channel blockers (verapamil or diltiazem). In some cases, cardioversion or electrophysiological ablation may be an option.

AV re-entry tachycardia

Conduction of impulses between the atria and the ventricles can normally only occur via one route, the AV node. However, some individuals have an additional connection between the atria and the ventricles, known as an *accessory pathway* (Figure 7.10).

The presence of an accessory pathway means that there are *two* distinct routes for conduction of impulses between atria and ventricles – via the AV node, as normal, but also via the

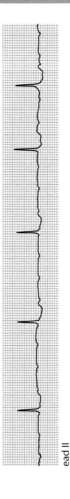

Lead II

Figure 7.9 Atrial tachycardia. There are inverted P waves (in lead II) indicating an atrial rhythm arising from near the AV node. The atrial rate is 167 beats/min. There is variable AV block, so the ventricular rhythm is irregular with a rate of 40–60 beats/min.

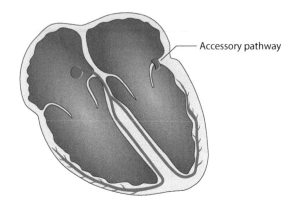

Figure 7.10 **Accessory pathway.** There is a left-sided accessory pathway between the left atrium and the left ventricle.

AV re-entry tachycardia (AVRT) can occur. In AVRT, an impulse can travel down one route and back up the other, to form a continuous re-entry circuit.

Most accessory pathways can conduct impulses *antegradely* (from atria to ventricles). When antegrade conduction occurs during normal sinus rhythm, *ventricular pre-excitation* is evident on the ECG, in the form of a *delta wave* (a slurred early upstroke of the QRS complex, Figure 7.11). In addition, because the accessory pathway conducts impulses very rapidly between atria and ventricles, lacking the intrinsic 'slowness' of the AV node, the *PR interval is short* (<0.12 s). However, once the wave of depolarization reaches the ventricular myocardium via the accessory pathway, it

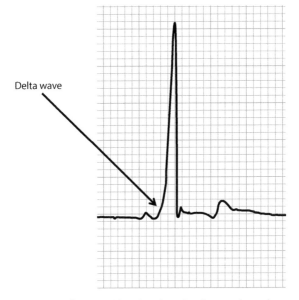

Delta wave

Figure 7.11 Delta wave. There is a slurred early upstroke to the QRS complex (a delta wave). Note that the PR interval is short.

His–Purkinje system. Instead, the impulse has to travel myocyte-to-myocyte, and because this is slower than normal the resulting QRS complex has a slow-rising 'slurred' initial upstroke. This is the delta wave of ventricular pre-excitation. Meanwhile, the wave of depolarization has *also* been travelling through the AV node, in the usual way, and when it reaches the His–Purkinje system, the rest of the

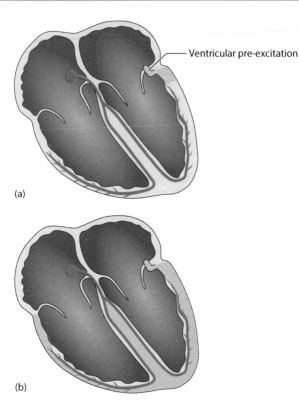

(a)

(b)

Figure 7.12 Ventricular pre-excitation. (a) There is early activation of part of the ventricular myocardium via the accessory pathway. (b) The remainder of the myocardium is depolarized in the normal way, via the AV node and the His–Purkinje system, shortly

Thus the slurred delta wave is followed by the rapid upstroke of an otherwise normal QRS complex.

When a short PR interval and delta wave are seen on an ECG, this is called a Wolff–Parkinson–White (WPW) *pattern*, and this is seen in approximately 0.2% of the general population (Figure 7.13). For most people, a WPW pattern on their ECG is simply an incidental finding, and the presence of an accessory pathway never leads to any arrhythmias. However, for some, it acts as a substrate for AVRT, and these patients are then said to have WPW *syndrome*.

AVRT in WPW syndrome

In 95% of episodes of AVRT in patients with WPW syndrome, the re-entry circuit travels down the AV node and back up the accessory pathway. This is known as an *orthodromic AVRT*, and is usually triggered by an atrial ectopic beat. An ECG during orthodromic AVRT (Figure 7.14) shows a regular narrow QRS complex tachycardia at a heart rate of 130–220 beats/min.

An inverted P wave is often visible after just each QRS complex, representing retrograde activation of the atria each time the impulse re-enters the atria via the accessory pathway.

Much less commonly (5% episodes), the re-entry circuit travels down the accessory pathway and back up through the AV node – this is an *antidromic AVRT*, and in this situation the QRS complexes are regular and *broad*. This occurs because the ventricles are depolarized

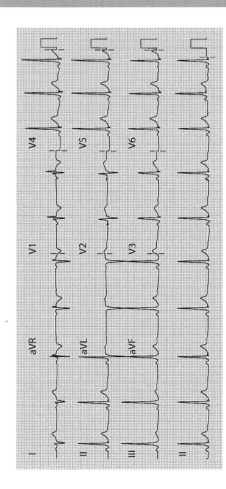

igure 7.13 Wolff–Parkinson–White pattern. The PR interval is short, and there is a slurred early pstroke to the QRS complex (a delta wave).

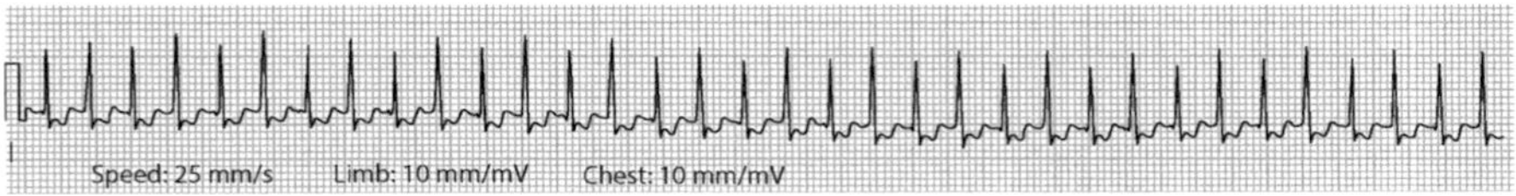

Speed: 25 mm/s   Limb: 10 mm/mV   Chest: 10 mm/mV

Lead II

Figure 7.14 Orthodromic atrioventricular re-entry tachycardia (AVRT). There is a regular narrow-complex tachycardia (204 beats/min) with inverted P waves (distorting the ST segments) following each QRS complex.

via the accessory pathway, which means the impulses can't gain access to the His–Purkinje system and the depolarization has to occur from myocyte-to-myocyte (as with the delta wave, see 'AV re-entry tachycardia' section). Antidromic AVRT can be difficult to distinguish from ventricular tachycardia.

ATRIAL FIBRILLATION IN WOLFF–PARKINSON–WHITE SYNDROME

AVRT is not the only arrhythmia that can occur in WPW syndrome. AF (or other atrial tachyarrhythmias, such as atrial flutter or atrial tachycardia) can occur, and are *potentially life-threatening* in this context because of the risk of very rapid ventricular rates. If a patient with an accessory pathway develops one of these atrial tachyarrhythmias, seek immediate advice from a cardiologist.

Termination of AVRT

An episode of AVRT can be terminated by blocking the AV node, thereby breaking the re-entry circuit. The *Valsalva manoeuvre* increases vagal inhibition of AV nodal conduction, thus slowing AV nodal conduction and terminating the tachycardia. Another option is for a trained clinician to perform *carotid sinus massage* (while monitoring the ECG) with the same aim, as long as the patient does not have carotid bruits or any history of cerebrovascular events.

VALSALVA MANOEUVRE

The Valsalva manoeuvre describes the action of forced expiration against a closed glottis. To perform it, patients should be asked to breathe in and then to strain for a few seconds with their breath held. Alternatively, they can be given a 20 mL plastic syringe and asked to 'blow' into the hole to try to push out the plunger from the opposite end. This is impossible to achieve, but in trying to do so the patient effectively performs a Valsalva manoeuvre.

Drug treatments to terminate an episode of AVRT include intravenous adenosine (contraindicated by asthma or obstructive airways disease) or intravenous verapamil (contraindicated if the patient has recently taken a beta blocker). If the patient is haemodynamically compromised, consider urgent DC cardioversion.

In the longer term, electrophysiological ablation of the accessory pathway is curative in a very high proportion of cases, at relatively low risk, and so should be considered a first-line therapy in symptomatic patients with WPW syndrome.

AV nodal re-entry tachycardia

AVNRT is, like AVRT, a tachycardia that is based around a re-entry circuit. However, the re-entry circuit of AVNRT occurs on a much smaller scale than in AVRT, occurring in the tissues within or just adjacent to the AV node. This is sometimes referred to as a micro re-entry circuit (as opposed to the macro re-entry circuit in AVRT).

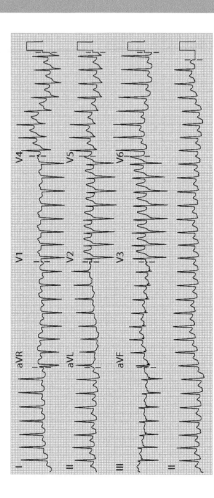

Figure 7.15 Atrioventricular nodal re-entry tachycardia (AVNRT). There is a regular narrow-complex tachycardia with a heart rate of 180 beats/min. P waves can just be discerned at the end of the QRS complexes in some of the leads.

With each circuit of the impulse, the atria and ventricles are depolarized simultaneously. As a result, the (inverted) P waves are buried within the QRS complexes and can be difficult or impossible to discern. The ECG shows a regular narrow complex tachycardia, with a ventricular rate usually 180–250 beats/min (Figure 7.15).

Distinguishing between AVNRT and AVRT can be difficult, although an ECG in sinus rhythm may help (as it may reveal evidence of ventricular pre-excitation, supporting a diagnosis of AVRT). The definitive diagnosis can prove challenging, however, and sometimes requires electrophysiological studies.

Treatment of AVNRT

As with AVRT (see 'AV re-entry tachycardia' section), an episode of AVNRT can be terminated by blocking the AV node, thereby breaking the cycle of electrical activity. For the prevention of recurrent episodes of AVNRT in the longer term for symptomatic patients, catheter ablation is the treatment of choice.

Further reading

Camm AJ, Lip GYH, De Caterina R et al. 2012 focused update of the ESC guidelines for the management of atrial fibrillation. *Eur Heart J* 2012; **33**: 2719–2747.

Whinnett ZI, Sohaib SMA, Davies DW. Diagnosis and management of supraventricular tachycardia. *BMJ* 2012; **345**: e7769.

Chapter 8

Ventricular rhythms

Ventricular rhythms are those which arise from the ventricles, that is below the level of the atrioventricular node. These include:

- Ventricular ectopic beats (VEBs)
- Accelerated idioventricular rhythm
- Monomorphic ventricular tachycardia (VT)
- Polymorphic VT
- Ventricular fibrillation (VF)

Ventricular ectopic beats

Like atrial ectopic beats (see Chapter 7), ventricular ectopic beats (VEBs) appear *earlier* than expected. VEBs are also called ventricular extrasystoles, ventricular premature complexes (VPCs), ventricular premature beats (VPBs) or premature ventricular contractions (PVCs). Isolated VEBs are common, occurring in 40%–75% of individuals during ambulatory ECG monitoring. The common causes are listed in Table 8.1.

Table 8.1 Common causes of ventricular ectopic beats

• Myocardial ischaemia/infarction
• Electrolyte disturbance (e.g. hypokalaemia, hypomagnesaemia)
• Myocarditis and cardiomyopathies
• Caffeine
• Alcohol
• Sympathomimetic drugs (e.g. salbutamol, dobutamine)

VEBs are identified by a QRS complex that is broad and appears earlier than expected (Figure 8.1). Because VEBs arise within the ventricular myocardium, the impulse cannot make use of the His–Purkinje rapid conduction system. As a result, conduction of the impulse has to occur slowly from myocyte to myocyte, and so ventricular depolarization is slower than usual, which is why the QRS complex is broad (>0.12 s).

VEBs are 'frequent' when they occur at a rate >60/h. Multiple VEBs which share the same QRS complex morphology originate from a single focus within the ventricles and are called *unifocal*. Where the VEBs have two or more different morphologies, they arise from different foci and are called *multifocal*.

There may be a regular pattern to the occurrence of VEBs: If every normal beat is followed by a VEB, the patient is said to be in *ventricular bigeminy* (Figure 8.2). If every third beat is a VEB, this is *ventricular trigeminy*, and if every fourth beat is a VEB, this is *ventricular quadrigeminy*. A pair of VEBs

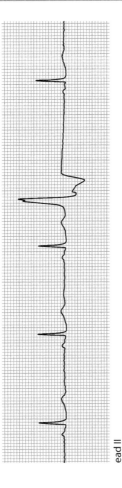

ead II

igure 8.1 Ventricular ectopic beat. After three normal sinus beats, there is a ventricular ectopic eat, followed by another normal sinus beat.

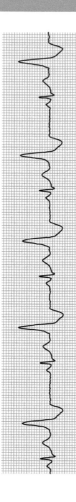

ead II

igure 8.2 Ventricular bigeminy. Every normal complex is followed by a ventricular ectopic beat.

occurring in succession is called a *ventricular couplet*. Three or more VEBs in succession is *ventricular tachycardia* (see 'Monomorphic ventricular tachycardia' section).

VEBs can be harmless, particularly when the heart is structurally normal, but can also be associated with more hazardous arrhythmias, especially when heart disease is present. VEBs can occur at the same time as the T wave of the preceding beat – such 'R on T' VEBs (Figure 8.3) can act as a trigger for VT or fibrillation.

Even though some VEBs can precipitate fatal arrhythmias, the routine treatment of incidental VEBs with anti-arrhythmic drugs has *not* been shown to decrease mortality. Some patients may be considerably troubled by symptoms caused by the VEBs and will benefit from using an anti-arrhythmic agent, as may patients who have experienced a potentially dangerous arrhythmia. Where feasible, electrophysiological ablation can be considered where symptoms are troublesome or there is a risk of malignant arrhythmias.

Accelerated idioventricular rhythm

Accelerated idioventricular rhythm is essentially a slow form of VT, with a heart rate of less than 120 beats/min (Figure 8.4). It occurs when an ectopic focus within the ventricles starts firing with a rate just higher than that of the sinoatrial node – this ventricular focus then takes over the cardiac rhythm.

It is most commonly seen in the context of myocardial reperfusion during the treatment of an acute myocardial infarction. Other causes include electrolyte abnormalities (which may require correction), myocarditis, cardiomyopathy

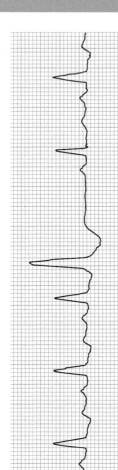

ead II

Figure 8.3 'R on T' ventricular ectopic beat. A ventricular ectopic beat occurs on the T wave of the third sinus beat.

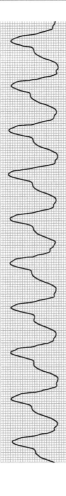

lead II

figure 8.4 Accelerated idioventricular rhythm. There is a broad complex (ventricular) rhythm with a rate of 88 beats/min.

Accelerated idioventricular rhythm is usually well tolerated and essentially 'benign' – it is not usually necessary to treat it with antiarrhythmic drugs (indeed, trying to suppress accelerated idioventricular rhythm can lead to disastrous decompensation).

Monomorphic ventricular tachycardia

VT is a *broad-complex tachycardia*, defined as three or more successive ventricular beats at a heart rate above 100 beats/min and with a QRS complex duration >0.12 s (Figure 8.5). VT arises most commonly as a re-entry circuit around an area of myocardial scarring (for instance, as a result of myocardial infarction). Other less common mechanisms include increased automaticity of a specific ventricular focus and abnormal triggering. Common causes of VT are listed in Table 8.2.

An episode of VT can be described as sustained or non-sustained. This is defined as follows:

- Non-sustained VT self-terminates in <30 s
- Sustained VT lasts >30 s (or requires urgent termination within 30 s due to haemodynamic compromise).

VT can also be classified as monomorphic or polymorphic:

- Monomorphic VT arises from a single ventricular focus and has a uniform QRS complex morphology
- Polymorphic VT has a changing ventricular focus and therefore has a varying QRS complex morphology.

Polymorphic VT is discussed in more detail in the 'Polymorphic ventricular tachycardia' section.

Sustained VT usually occurs at a heart rate of 150–250 beats/min, but this can be well tolerated and may not cause haemodynamic disturbances. Do *not* assume, therefore, that

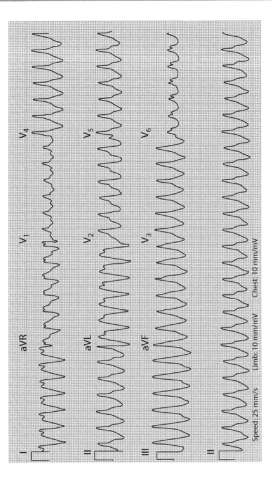

Figure 8.5 Ventricular tachycardia. There is a broad complex tachycardia with a rate of 52 beats/min. The QRS complex duration is 0.164 s.

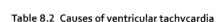

Table 8.2 Causes of ventricular tachycardia

• Myocardial ischaemia and infarction
• Cardiomyopathy
• Myocarditis
• Congenital heart disease (repaired or unrepaired)
• Electrolyte disturbances
• Pro-arrhythmic drugs
• Right ventricular outflow tract tachycardia
• Long QT syndrome
• Brugada syndrome

The symptoms of VT can vary from mild palpitations to dizziness, syncope and cardiac arrest.

The urgency and type of treatment required depends upon the clinical state of the patient. When a patient has pulseless VT, they are in cardiac arrest and should be managed in accordance with the adult advanced life support algorithm (Figure 8.6). Where a patient with VT has a pulse, they should be managed in line with the Adult Tachycardia (With Pulse) algorithm (Figure 5.7).

Following the initial management and correction of VT, longer-term management should be discussed with a cardiologist. Long-term prophylaxis is usually not necessary for VT occurring within the first 48 h following an acute myocardial infarction. Where prophylaxis is needed, effective drug treatments include sotalol (particularly when VT is exercise related) or amiodarone. VT related to bradycardia

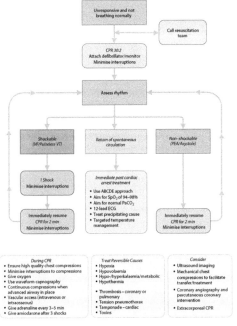

Figure 8.6 Resuscitation Council (UK) 2015 adult advanced life support algorithm. ABCDE, Airway, Breathing, Circulation, Disability, Exposure (see 'How is the patient?' section in Chapter 6); CPR, cardiopulmonary resuscitation; PEA, pulseless electrical activity; VF, ventricular fibrillation; VT, ventricular tachycardia. (Reproduced with the kind permission of the Resuscitation Council, London, UK, *Resuscitation Guidelines 2015*, https://www.resus.org.uk/resuscitation-guidelines/adult-advanced-life-support/ accessed 18 October 2015.)

to remove a ventricular focus or re-entry circuit identified by electrophysiological testing. Finally, an implantable cardioverter-defibrillator can be implanted to deliver overdrive pacing and/or shocks for recurrent episodes of VT and VF.

VT can be idiopathic in the context of an apparently structurally normal heart – in this context, the most common type is right ventricular outflow tract (RVOT) tachycardia, which accounts for around 10% of all forms of VT. The prognosis for these patients is generally good. It is important, however, not to mistake the relatively benign RVOT form of VT with VT caused by arrhythmogenic right ventricular cardiomyopathy (ARVC), which has a more sinister prognosis. In ARVC, the heart is *not* structurally normal, and the abnormal right ventricular morphology can be identified by echocardiography or cardiac magnetic resonance imaging. VT in the context of ARVC is treated with an ICD, whereas symptomatic RVOT tachycardia is usually treated with ablation.

BRUGADA SYNDROME

Be careful not to miss Brugada syndrome in patients presenting with ventricular arrhythmias, including VT and VF. The heart appears structurally normal in this condition, but the presence of an abnormality of the cardiac sodium channel predisposes to potentially lethal arrhythmias. Brugada syndrome is characterized on the ECG by a right bundle branch block morphology and persistent ST segment elevation in leads V1–V3. Patients with this ECG appearance need urgent assessment by a cardiologist.

Is this VT or SVT with aberrant conduction?

As we learnt in Chapter 6, a broad-complex tachycardia can have two possible explanations:

1. The tachycardia may be ventricular in origin (VT)
2. The tachycardia may be supraventricular in origin, but have a broad-complex rather than narrow-complex appearance because of a coexistent conduction problem, such as a bundle branch block (SVT *with aberrant conduction*).

The distinction between VT and SVT with aberrant conduction is not always straightforward. However, the distinction is important as the management of the two conditions is different (although in an emergency both VT and SVT usually respond to electrical cardioversion). When the diagnosis is unclear, the golden rule is as follows:

THE GOLDEN RULE

A broad-complex tachycardia is always assumed to be VT unless proven otherwise.

Most cases (80%) of broad complex tachycardia are due to VT, and the likelihood of VT (rather than SVT with aberrant conduction) is even higher when structural heart disease is present. Haemodynamic stability is not a reliable guide in distinguishing between VT and SVT with aberrant conduction, as VT can be remarkably well tolerated by some patients.

A very reliable ECG indicator of VT is the presence of *atrioventricular dissociation*, where the atria and ventricles are seen to be working independently. Unfortunately, such features are seen in fewer than half of the cases of VT, so the absence of independent atrial activity does not exclude VT as a diagnosis. Atrioventricular dissociation is indicated by the following:

Independent P wave activity, as shown by the presence of P waves occurring at a slower rate than the QRS complexes and bearing no relation to them (Figure 8.7).

Fusion beats, which appear when the ventricles are activated by an atrial impulse and a ventricular impulse arriving simultaneously (Figure 8.8).

Capture beats, which occur when an atrial impulse manages to 'capture' the ventricles for a beat, causing a normal QRS complex, which may be preceded by a normal P wave (Figure 8.9).

Other ECG features can also provide clues to the diagnosis. Most patients with SVT and aberrant conduction will have a QRS complex morphology that looks like a typical LBBB or RBBB pattern. Patients with VT will often (but not always) have more unusual-looking QRS complexes which don't fit a typical bundle branch block pattern.

Many other ECG features suggest (but do not prove) a diagnosis of VT rather than SVT with aberrant conduction, including:

- Very broad QRS complexes (>160 ms)
- Extreme QRS axis deviation
- Concordance (same QRS direction) in leads V1–V6
- An interval >100 ms from the start of the R wave to the deepest point of the S wave in one chest lead (this is called Brugada's sign)
- A notch in the downstroke of the S wave (this is called Josephson's sign).

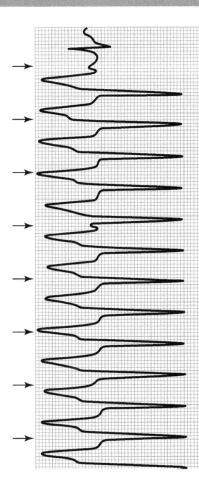

Lead II

Figure 8.7 Independent P wave activity. There is a broad-complex tachycardia (VT). The arrows show independent P waves deforming the QRS complexes. The last beat is a capture beat.

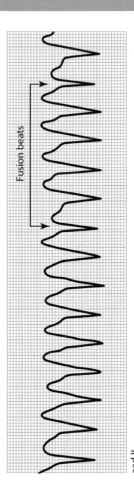

Lead II

Figure 8.8 Fusion beats. There is a broad-complex tachycardia (VT). The arrows show fusion beats.

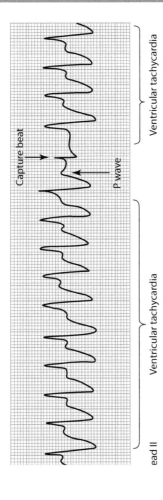

Figure 8.9 Capture beats. There is a broad-complex tachycardia (VT). There is one normal QRS complex (capture beat).

Polymorphic ventricular tachycardia

In contrast to monomorphic VT, polymorphic VT is distinguished by a *varying* QRS complex morphology (Figure 8.10). Like monomorphic VT, polymorphic VT can be classified as sustained or non-sustained. Polymorphic VT falls into two distinct categories based upon the duration of the QT interval (measured during sinus rhythm):

- Polymorphic VT in the setting of a normal QT interval
- Polymorphic VT in the setting of a prolonged QT interval

When the underlying QT interval is normal, polymorphic VT may be due to myocardial ischaemia/infarction, coronary reperfusion (following myocardial infarction), structural heart disease or the rare condition of catecholaminergic polymorphic VT.

When polymorphic VT is seen in the context of a prolonged QT interval, it is commonly called *torsades de pointes* ('twisting of the points'). There are several causes of QT interval prolongation, including hypocalcaemia, acute myocarditis, long QT syndrome and certain drugs. QT interval prolongation is discussed further in Chapter 13. Polymorphic VT carries a risk of triggering VF and so urgent assessment is warranted. In an emergency, standard adult life support protocols (Figures 5.7 and 8.6) should be followed. Treat underlying causes, such as myocardial ischaemia/ infarction or electrolyte abnormalities, and stop any causative drugs. If the underlying QT interval is prolonged, useful measures can also include the administration of intravenous magnesium and consideration of temporary transvenous pacing (which increases the heart rate and thereby shortens the QT interval). In the longer term, an

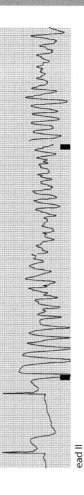

ead II

figure 8.10 Polymorphic ventricular tachycardia. This patient presented with an inferior T-segment elevation myocardial infarction. An 'R on T' ventricular ectopic beat triggers entricular tachycardia with a continuously varying QRS complex morphology.

Lead II

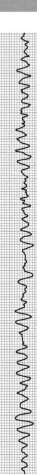

Figure 8.11 Ventricular fibrillation. This rhythm strip demonstrates the chaotic rhythm of ventricular fibrillation.

ICD may be required if the patient is judged to be at high risk of recurrent arrhythmias and sudden cardiac death.

Ventricular fibrillation

In VF, the ECG shows a chaotic rhythm without clearly discernible P waves, QRS complexes or T waves (Figure 8.11). Untreated VF is a rapidly fatal arrhythmia. It therefore requires immediate diagnosis and treatment according to the adult advanced life support algorithm (Figure 8.6). Causes of VF are listed in Table 8.3. Always check for reversible causes following an episode of VF. In the longer term, an ICD should be considered for survivors of VF who are considered to be at risk of recurrent VF. Such patients may also require appropriate antiarrhythmic medication (e.g. amiodarone, beta blockers) to reduce the risk of recurrence.

Table 8.3 Causes of ventricular fibrillation

• Myocardial ischaemia/infarction
• Cardiomyopathy
• Myocarditis
• Electrolyte disturbances
• Pro-arrhythmic drugs
• Long QT syndrome
• Brugada syndrome
• Cardiac trauma
• Electrical shock

Further reading

Alzand BSN, Crijns HJGM. Diagnostic criteria of broad QRS complex tachycardia: Decades of evolution. *Europace* 2011; **13**: 465–472.

Jastrzebski M, Kukla P, Czarnecka D et al. Comparison of five electrocardiographic methods for differentiation of wide QRS-complex tachycardias. *Europace* 2012; **14**: 1165–1171.

Ng GA. Treating patients with ventricular ectopic beats. *Heart* 2006; **92**: 1707–1712.

Chapter 9

Conduction problems and types of block

The normal conduction of impulses from the sinoatrial (SA) node to the ventricles was described in Chapter 1 – an impulse arises with spontaneous depolarization of the SA node, which then depolarizes the atria before reaching the atrioventricular (AV) node. The impulse then passes via the bundle of His to reach the left and right bundle branches, before depolarizing the ventricular myocardium via the Purkinje fibres (Figure 1.5).

Problems with conduction can occur at four key points in this pathway:

1. SA node
2. AV node
3. Left or right bundle branches
4. Left anterior or posterior fascicles

Conduction problems at the SA node

If impulses are blocked from exiting the SA node, SA block is the result. Because the impulse cannot leave the SA

P waves are missing (Figure 9.1). SA block requires pacing if it is causing symptoms.

In SA block, the SA node itself *does* depolarize, but the impulse does not reach the rest of the atria. The intrinsic rhythm of the SA node is maintained, so when the SA block resolves and a P wave finally does appear, it appears exactly 'on time' – by mapping out the spacing between the earlier P waves, and marking where the missing P waves should have occurred, you can show that when the P wave reappears, the regular rhythm of the SA node has been maintained throughout the period of SA block.

Conduction problems at the AV node

When there are conduction problems at the AV node (or just below the AV node, in the bundle of His), conduction of impulses between the atria and ventricles is affected. This can take several forms or 'degrees'.

First-degree AV block

In first-degree AV block, conduction through the AV node is slower than usual and the PR interval is therefore prolonged. Nonetheless, every P wave is followed by a QRS complex and therefore there are no 'dropped' beats.

The normal PR interval is 0.12–0.20 s, and so first-degree AV block is diagnosed when the PR interval measures >0.20 s (Figure 9.2). First-degree AV block is a common feature of vagally induced bradycardia, as an increase in vagal tone decreases AV nodal conduction. It may also be a feature of

- Drugs (e.g. beta blockers, verapamil, diltiazem)
- Electrolyte abnormalities

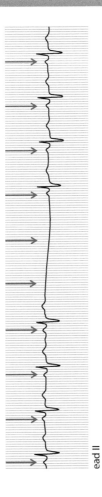

Lead II

Figure 9.1 SA block. The P waves are marked by arrows. There are two missing P waves as a result of SA block, but the next P wave appears exactly where it was predicted. The SA node has therefore continued to depolarize, maintaining its cycle, but two of its impulses were blocked from depolarizing the atria.

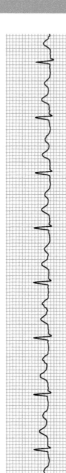

Lead II

Figure 9.2 First-degree AV block. The PR interval is prolonged at 0.28 s.

- Ischaemic heart disease
- Lyme disease

Second-degree AV block

In second-degree AV block, there is an intermittent failure of AV conduction and as a result some P waves are not followed by QRS complexes. There are two types of second-degree AV block:

1. If the PR interval gradually lengthens with each beat, until one P wave fails to produce a QRS complex, the patient has *Mobitz type I AV block*.
2. If the PR interval is fixed and normal, but occasionally a P wave fails to produce a QRS complex, the patient has *Mobitz type II AV block*.

Mobitz type I AV block (Figure 9.3), also known as the Wenckebach phenomenon, is usually a consequence of conduction problems within the AV node itself, sometimes simply as a result of high vagal tone – for instance, it is more commonly seen during sleep and has a higher prevalence in athletes.

One can imagine Mobitz type I AV block as the AV node becoming increasingly 'tired' as it conducts each P wave – as a result, the node takes longer and longer to conduct each subsequent P wave until it totally 'gives up' and fails to conduct a P wave at all. This however gives the AV node a chance to 'rest', and by the time the next P wave arrives it is ready to conduct normally, before the cycle repeats itself.

Mobitz type II AV block (Figure 9.4) is usually a consequence of conduction problems distal to the AV node (infranodal). As a result, there is a higher risk of progression to

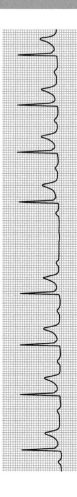

Lead II

Figure 9.3 Mobitz type I AV block (Wenckebach phenomenon). The PR interval gradually lengthens until a P wave fails to be conducted. The PR interval resets, and the cycle repeats.

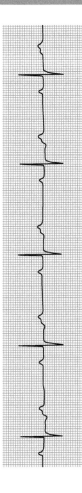

ead II

igure 9.4 Mobitz type II AV block. There is intermittent failure of P waves to be conducted to
e ventricles, with no lengthening of the PR interval.

third-degree AV block and the prognosis is therefore worse than for Mobitz type I AV block.

PACING IN SECOND-DEGREE AV BLOCK

Mobitz type II AV block requires pacing regardless of symptoms. Pacing for Mobitz type I AV block is more debatable, but is certainly indicated if the patient has symptomatic bradycardia or pauses.

Third-degree AV block

In third-degree AV block ('complete heart block'), there is complete interruption of conduction between atria and ventricles, so that the two are working independently. The possible causes are listed in Table 9.1.

In third-degree AV block QRS complexes usually arise as the result of a ventricular escape rhythm (see Chapter 9), in which the QRS complexes are usually broad and the ventricular rate is typically 15–40 beats/min. However if the level of AV block is located in or just below the AV node, a junctional escape rhythm may arise with narrow QRS complexes and a ventricular rate around 40–60 beats/min (Figure 9.5).

Third-degree AV block requires pacing regardless of symptoms.

Block at the bundle branches

Moving down the conducting system beyond the bundle of His, *bundle branch block* can affect either the left or right

Table 9.1 Causes of third-degree atrioventricular block

• Congenital
• Acquired
• Drug toxicity (e.g. antiarrhythmics, donepezil)
• Fibrosis/calcification of the conduction system
• Myocardial ischaemia/infarction
• Infection (e.g. Lyme disease)
• Myocardial infiltration (e.g. amyloid, sarcoid)
• Neuromuscular diseases (e.g. myotonic muscular dystrophy)
• Metabolic disorders (e.g. hypothyroidism)
• Cardiac procedures (e.g. ablation procedures, aortic valve surgery)

branches are blocked, this is equivalent to third-degree AV block, as no impulses will be able to reach the ventricular myocardium from the atria.

Left bundle branch block

In left bundle branch block (LBBB), there is a failure of conduction down the left bundle, and so the left ventricle cannot be depolarized in the normal way via its Purkinje fibres. However, the right ventricle can still depolarize normally via the still-functioning right bundle. The right ventricle therefore depolarizes normally, but then this wave of depolarization has to spread slowly across to the left ventricle, going from myocyte to myocyte, until the left

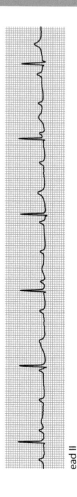

ead II

igure 9.5 Third-degree AV block. There is a complete block of AV conduction, with sinus rhythm

n the atria and a narrow complex ('junctional') escape rhythm in the ventricles.

This delay in left ventricular activation causes *interventricular dyssynchrony*, with the right ventricle depolarizing (and contracting) before the left ventricle, which reduces the efficiency of cardiac function. In some patients with heart failure and LBBB, symptoms (and prognosis) can be improved by re-synchronizing the ventricles using a cardiac resynchronization therapy (CRT) pacemaker.

The ECG in LBBB has an appearance as shown in Figure 9.6, with broad QRS complexes (due to the prolonged process of depolarization) and characteristic morphologies to the QRS complexes. This is commonly referred to as a 'W' shape to the QRS complex in lead V1, and an 'M' shape in lead V6.

WHAT CAUSES THE SHAPE OF THE QRS COMPLEXES IN LBBB?

In LBBB, the interventricular septum has to depolarize from right to left, a reversal of the normal pattern. This causes a small Q wave in lead V1 and a small R wave in lead V6. The right ventricle is depolarized normally via the right bundle branch, causing an R wave in lead V1 and an S wave in lead V6. Then, the left ventricle is depolarized by the right, causing an S wave in lead V1 and another R wave (called R') in lead V6. This gives the QRS complexes in LBBB their characteristic 'W' shape in lead V1 and an 'M' shape in lead V6.

The presence of LBBB is almost invariably an indication of underlying pathology (Table 9.2), and the patient should be

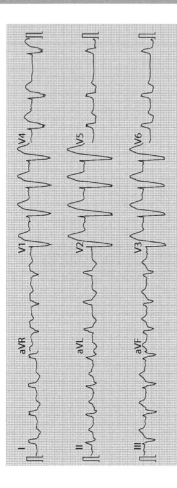

Figure 9.6 Left bundle branch block. There are broad QRS complexes, with a QRS complex morphology as explained in text. The underlying rhythm in this case happens to be atrial fibrillation.

Table 9.2 Causes of left bundle branch block

• Ischaemic heart disease
• Cardiomyopathy
• Left ventricular hypertrophy
• Hypertension
• Aortic stenosis
• Fibrosis of the conduction system

The presence of LBBB makes interpretation of the ECG beyond the QRS complex extremely challenging. As a result, it can be very difficult to recognize previous myocardial infarction in a patient with pre-existing LBBB. However, the Sgarbossa criteria can help. This is a scoring system for identifying acute myocardial infarction in the presence of LBBB (or a paced rhythm) on the ECG. There are three criteria:

1. ST segment elevation ≥1 mm and concordant with QRS complex (5 points)
2. ST segment depression ≥1 mm in lead V1, V2 or V3 (3 points)
3. ST segment elevation ≥5 mm and discordant with QRS complex (2 points)

A score of ≥3 points has a high specificity (but low sensitivity) for acute moycardial infarction in the setting of LBBB.

Right bundle branch block

In contrast with LBBB, RBBB is a relatively common finding

Table 9.3 Causes of right bundle branch block

• Normal variant
• Ischaemic heart disease
• Cardiomyopathy
• Atrial septal defect
• Ebstein's anomaly
• Pulmonary embolism (usually massive)

underlying disease (Table 9.3) and should be investigated according to the clinical presentation.

In right bundle branch block (RBBB), there is a failure of conduction down the right bundle, and so the right ventricle cannot be depolarized in the normal way via its Purkinje fibres. However, the left ventricle can still depolarize normally via the still-functioning left bundle. The left ventricle therefore depolarizes normally, but then this wave of depolarization has to spread slowly across to the right ventricle, going from myocyte to myocyte, until the right ventricle has also depolarized. As with LBBB, this delay in right ventricular activation causes interventricular dyssynchrony.

The ECG in RBBB has an appearance as shown in Figure 9.7, with broad QRS complexes (due to the prolonged process of depolarization) and characteristic morphologies to the QRS complexes. This is commonly referred to as an 'M' shape to the QRS complex in lead V1, and a 'W' shape in lead V6.

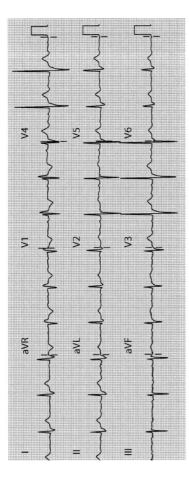

Figure 9.7 Right bundle branch block. There are broad QRS complexes, with a QRS complex morphology as explained in text.

WHAT CAUSES THE SHAPE OF THE QRS COMPLEXES IN RBBB?

In RBBB, the interventricular septum depolarizes normally, from left to right, causing a tiny R wave in lead V1 and a small 'septal' Q wave in lead V6. The left ventricle is depolarized normally via the left bundle branch, causing an S wave in lead V1 and an R wave in lead V6. Then, the right ventricle is depolarized by the left, causing another R wave (called R') in lead V1 and an S wave in lead V6. This gives the QRS complexes in RBBB their characteristic 'M' shape in lead V1 and a 'W' shape in lead V6.

AN AIDE-MÉMOIRE

The name 'William Marrow' should help you remember:

In LBBB, the QRS looks like a 'W' in lead V1 and an 'M' in lead V6 (William).

In RBBB, the QRS looks like an 'M' in lead V1 and a 'W' in lead V6 (Marrow).

Block at the fascicles

The left bundle does not have to be blocked in its entirety. Instead, just one of its fascicles (anterior or posterior) may become blocked (Figure 1.5). When this occurs, it is known as a fascicular block (or 'hemiblock').

Left anterior fascicular block

Block of the anterior fascicle of the left bundle branch is known as left anterior fascicular block (LAFB). On the ECG, the primary consequence of LAFB is left axis deviation (where the QRS axis lies beyond −30° – see

LAFB can result from fibrosis of the conducting system (of any cause) or from myocardial infarction. On its own, it is not thought to carry any prognostic significance.

Left posterior fascicular block

Block of the posterior fascicle of the left bundle branch is known as left posterior fascicular block (LPFB), and this is much less common than LAFB. On the ECG, the primary consequence of LPFB is right axis deviation (where the QRS axis lies beyond +90° – see Chapter 2).

BIFASCICULAR AND TRIFASCICULAR BLOCK

Left anterior or posterior fascicular block in combination with right bundle branch block (see Chapter 9) means that two of the three main conducting pathways to the ventricles are blocked. This is termed *bifascicular block*.

Block of the conducting pathways can occur in any combination (Table 9.4). A block of both fascicles is the equivalent of left bundle branch block. Block of the right bundle branch and either fascicle is a bifascicular block. If a bifascicular block is combined with first-degree AV block (long PR interval), it is called a *trifascicular block*.

Block of the right bundle branch and *both* fascicles leaves no route for impulses to reach the ventricles, and this is the equivalent of third-degree AV block (see 'Block at the bundle branches' section in Chapter 9).

A bifascicular or trifascicular block in a patient with syncopal episodes is often sufficient indication for a permanent pacemaker, even if higher degrees of block have not been documented. An *asymptomatic* bifascicular block, or even trifascicular block, is not necessarily an indication for pacing.

Table 9.4 Combinations of conduction blocks

Conduction abnormalities can occur in different permutations:
LAFB + LPFB = LBBB
RBBB + LAFB = Bifascicular block
RBBB + LPFB = Bifascicular block
RBBB + LAFB + 1st degree AV block = trifascicular block
RBBB + LPFB + 1st degree AV block = trifascicular block
RBBB + LBBB = third-degree AV block ('complete heart block')
RBBB + LAFB + LPFB = third-degree AV block ('complete heart block')

Escape rhythms

Escape rhythms act as a 'safety net' for the heart and appear when there is a failure of normal impulse generation or conduction. Without escape rhythms, a complete failure of impulse generation or conduction would lead to ventricular asystole and death. Instead, the heart has a number of 'backup' pacemakers that can take over if normal impulse generation or conduction fails. The subsidiary pacemakers are located in the AV junction (AV node/bundle of His) and in the ventricular myocardium.

If the AV junction fails to receive impulses from the SA node (e.g. as a result of SA block), it will take over as the cardiac pacemaker. The QRS complexes generated will have the same morphology as normal, but at a slower rate of around 40–60 beats/min. Figure 9.5 shows third-degree heart block (at the level of the AV node) with a junctional (narrow complex) escape rhythm which, because the QRS complexes are narrow, must be arising 'high up' in the conduction system, that is at or just below the AV node. The AV junctional pacemaker will continue until it again starts to be inhibited by impulses from the SA node. If the AV junctional pacemaker itself fails, or its impulses are blocked, a ventricular pacemaker will take over. Its rhythm is even slower, at 15–40 beats/min, and the QRS complexes are broad because, arising within the ventricles, they cannot gain access to the Purkinje fibres and so conduction occurs slowly from myocyte to myocyte.

Further reading

The Task Force on Cardiac Pacing and Cardiac Resynchronization Therapy of the European Society of Cardiology (ESC). 2013 ESC Guidelines on cardiac pacing and cardiac resynchronization therapy. *Eur Heart J* 2013; **34**: 2281–2329.

QRS complexes and left ventricular hypertrophy

The QRS complex corresponds to depolarization of the ventricles. The Q wave is defined as the first negative deflection of the QRS complex, and corresponds to the depolarization of the interventricular septum. The septum normally depolarizes from left to right – this causes a small negative deflection in those leads that look at the heart from the left (I, aVL, V5 and V6) and therefore see the septal depolarization moving away from them (Figure 10.1). After the Q wave comes the RS portion of the QRS complex, corresponding to the depolarization of the rest of the ventricular myocardium.

Q wave

As already described, normally a small Q wave is seen in leads I, aVL, V5 and V6. A small Q wave may also be normal in lead III, and is often associated with an inverted T wave. Both may disappear on deep inspiration. Q waves can also be normal in lead aVR.

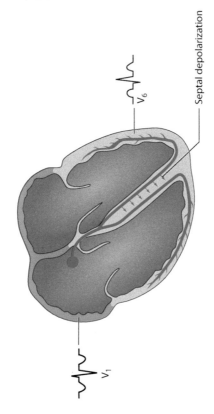

figure 10.1 Septal depolarization. The left-to-right depolarization of the interventricular septum causes small Q waves in the leads that look at the heart from the left.

Septal depolarization

Q waves in other leads are likely to be abnormal or 'pathological', particularly if they are

- >2 small squares deep, or
- >25% of the height of the following R wave in depth, and/or
- >1 small square wide

The presence of such 'pathological' Q waves indicates a region of myocardial damage/scarring, usually as a consequence of a myocardial infarction (Figure 10.2).

Tall QRS complexes

The height of the R wave and depth of the S wave vary from lead to lead in the normal ECG (as Figure 10.3 shows). As a rule, in the normal ECG

- The R wave *increases* in height from lead V1 to V5.
- The R wave is *smaller* than the S wave in leads V1 and V2.
- The R wave is *bigger* than the S wave in leads V5 and V6.
- The tallest R wave does not exceed 25 mm in height.
- The deepest S wave does not exceed 25 mm in depth.

Always look carefully at the R and S waves in each lead and check whether they conform to these criteria. If not, check whether the ECG calibration is correct (should be 1 mV = 10 mm). If the calibration is correct, consider whether the patient may have one of the following:

- Left ventricular hypertrophy (LVH)
- Right ventricular hypertrophy (RVH)

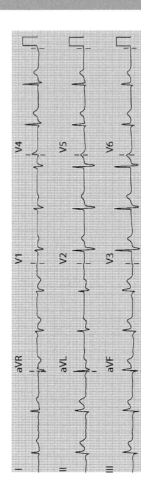

Figure 10.2 Inferior myocardial infarction (after 1 year). Pathological Q waves are present in leads II, III and aVF.

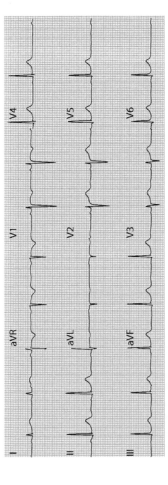

Figure 10.3 Normal 12-lead ECG. The size of the normal QRS complex varies from lead to lead.

Left ventricular hypertrophy

LVH occurs when the left ventricular myocardium thickens (hypertrophies) secondary to pressure overload. Common causes for pressure overload include high blood pressure and aortic stenosis (narrowing of the valve between the left ventricle and the aorta). LVH is also a key feature of hypertrophic cardiomyopathy (a genetic abnormality of the heart muscle).

Hypertrophy of the left ventricle causes tall R waves in the leads that 'look at' the left ventricle – I, aVL, V5 and V6 – and the reciprocal ('mirror image') change of deep S waves in leads that 'look at' the right ventricle – V1 and V2 (Figure 10.4).

There are many criteria for the ECG diagnosis of LVH, with varying sensitivity and specificity. Generally, the diagnostic criteria are quite specific (if the criteria are present, the likelihood of the patient having LVH is >90%), but not sensitive (the criteria will fail to detect 40%–80% of patients with LVH).

The simplest criteria to remember are the Sokolow–Lyon criteria, in which LVH is indicated by

- R wave >11 mm in lead aVL

or

- Sum of S wave in lead V1 plus the tallest R wave in either lead V5 or V6 >35 mm

If one (or both) of these criteria is met then the patient is said to have LVH by voltage criteria (not all patients who have apparent LVH on an ECG will have the diagnosis confirmed on further investigation by, for example, echocardiography). Any patient who has a suspicion of

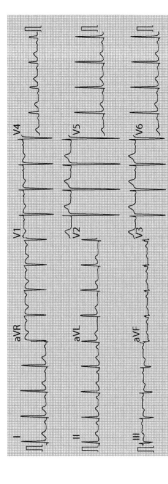

Figure 10.4 Left ventricular hypertrophy. Tall R waves in leads I, aVL, V5 and V6, with deep S waves in leads V1, V2 and V3.

LVH by voltage criteria on their ECG should have further investigation to rule out possible cardiomyopathy.

If there is evidence of LVH on the ECG, there may also be evidence of 'strain' (Figure 10.5), as evidenced by co-existent ST segment depression and/or T wave inversion (see Chapter 11).

Right ventricular hypertrophy

The pathophysiology of RVH is very similar to that of LVH. However, it is much less common. Causes of RVH include pulmonary hypertension, pulmonary stenosis, pulmonary embolism, chronic pulmonary disease (cor pulmonale) and congenital heart disease (Tetralogy of Fallot).

RVH may be recognized if the patient has a normal QRS complex duration (hence no bundle branch block) and:

- Right axis deviation (negative QRS in lead I and positive QRS in lead II)
- R wave in V1 is ≥6 mm in height
- A dominant S wave of ≥6 mm in depth in either V5 or V6

An example of RVH is shown in the ECG in Figure 10.6.

Small QRS complexes

Small QRS complexes indicate that relatively little of the voltage generated by ventricular depolarization is reaching the ECG electrodes. Although criteria exist for the normal upper limit of QRS complex size, there are no similar guidelines for the lower limit of QRS size and so this is based upon an 'eyeball' assessment.

Small QRS complexes may simply reflect a variant of normal. However, always check for incorrect ECG

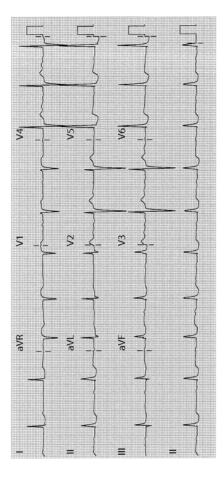

Figure 10.5 Left ventricular hypertrophy with 'strain'. There are tall R waves and deep S waves, with wave inversion in leads V5–V6.

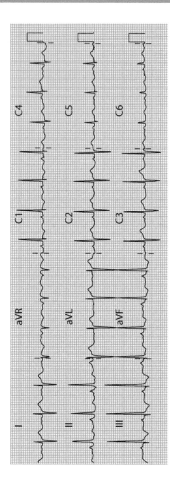

Figure 10.6 Right ventricular hypertrophy. There is a dominant R wave in lead V1, together with right axis deviation.

calibration (should be 1 mV = 10 mm). Also check whether the patient has obesity or emphysema – both of these conditions increase the distance between the heart and the chest electrodes.

However, if the QRS complexes appear small, and particularly if they have changed in relation to earlier ECG recordings, always consider the possibility of a pericardial effusion. This can be confirmed by echocardiography.

Broad QRS complexes

Normally the ventricles depolarize rapidly thanks to the rapid spread of the ventricular impulse via the His–Purkinje conduction system. As a result, the QRS complex duration (width) is <120 ms (i.e. the QRS complex is less than three small squares across).

If a QRS complex is broader than this, this indicates that the ventricles have depolarized slowly because the impulse has not been able to use the His–Purkinje system normally (Figure 10.7). This can occur because:

1. Part of the normal conduction system is not working, so the impulse cannot make full use of the rapidly conducting His–Purkinje system – this is what happens in left or right bundle branch block.

Or

2. The impulse has arisen within the ventricles to begin with, so it cannot get access into the His–Purkinje system via the atrioventricular node – this is what happens with ventricular ectopic beats, ventricular tachycardia and ventricular pacing.

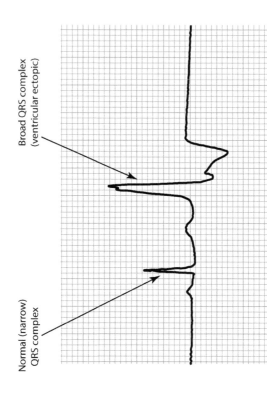

Broad QRS complex
(ventricular ectopic)

Normal (narrow)
QRS complex

Figure 10.7 Narrow and broad QRS complexes. A narrow QRS complex (normal) is followed by broad QRS complex (ventricular ectopic beat).

We cover left and right bundle branch blocks in more detail in the 'Block at the bundle branches' section in Chapter 9. We describe ventricular ectopic beats and ventricular tachycardia in Chapter 8.

Ventricular pacing

If the heart's electrical system starts to malfunction, then the patient may undergo implantation of a pacemaker. In summary, there are two main types of pacemaker: those that pace the atrium and those that pace the ventricles (many pacemakers will be capable of doing both).

Pacemakers work by replacing the natural wiring of the heart with an artificial system that has two main components: a generator box that generates the electrical current and wires that connect the generator box to the heart. Pacing is most commonly observed on the ECG as pacing 'spikes'. If it is an atrial pacemaker, these spikes will be visible just before the P wave, and if it is a ventricular pacemaker then the spikes will occur just before the QRS complex.

In most cases a ventricular pacing wire is placed in the right ventricle. This means that when the ventricle is paced, the impulse from the pacemaker is unable to make use of the His–Purkinje system (because an impulse can only do that if it travels to the ventricles via the atrioventricular node). As a result, paced ventricles depolarize slowly from myocyte-to-myocyte, with the right ventricle depolarizing before the left ventricle. Ventricular pacing spikes are therefore followed by a broad QRS complex, with a left bundle branch block appearance (Figure 10.8).

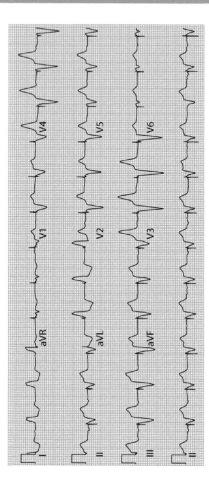

Figure 10.8 Ventricular pacing. Ventricular pacing spikes are followed by broad QRS complexes.

PACING 'ON DEMAND'

The most common reason the authors get contacted for advice about pacemakers is the belief that the pacemaker is not working, as no pacing spikes can be seen on the ECG. Generally, the absence of spikes indicates that the pacemaker is working 'on demand'. Thus, if the pacemaker is set at to pace the heart at 60 beats/min but the patient's natural heart rate is 70 beats/min, then no pacing spikes will be seen as the pacemaker is designed only to pace when it needs to. If the patient's heart rate rises above the minimum pacing rate, then the pacemaker will simply monitor the heart but will not need to do any pacing until the patient's heart rate falls back below the set pacing rate again. Most pacemakers do not need to pace all the time, and only do so when the patient is bradycardic. This avoids the need for unnecessary pacing and helps prolong the device's battery life.

Further reading

Bauml MA, Underwood DA. Left ventricular hypertrophy: An overlooked cardiovascular risk factor. *Cleveland Clinic J Med* 2010; **77**: 381–387.

Francia P, Balla C, Paneni F et al. Left bundle-branch block – Pathophysiology, prognosis, and clinical management. *Clin Cardiol* 2007; **30**: 110–115.

Chapter 11

ST segment elevation and depression

ST segment refers to the portion of the ECG that lies between the end of the S wave and the start of the T wave (Figure 2.5). It is a region of the ECG that needs careful assessment, as abnormalities of the ST segment can indicate acute cardiac problems such as myocardial ischaemia ('angina') or myocardial infarction ('heart attack').

You can also see ST segment changes with inflammation of the external lining of the heart (pericarditis). ST segment changes are also seen in association with other ECG abnormalities, such as left bundle branch block and Brugada syndrome. In this chapter, we describe how the ECG looks in each of these conditions, and explain how to tell the difference between them.

Assessing the ST segment

The ST segment can become elevated or depressed. Normally, the ST segment lies at the same level as (i.e. is 'isoelectric' with) the rest of the baseline of the

ECG (Figure 11.1). ST segment elevation occurs when the ST segment lies above the isoelectric (normal) baseline and ST segment depression when it lies below the isoelectric baseline.

To establish the isoelectric baseline place a straight line (a ruler or the edge of a sheet of paper will do) from the bottom of one of the P waves to the bottom of the next P wave on the ECG. This line represents the isoelectric baseline. Normally, the ST segment should be level with this line. Caution should be used when establishing the isoelectric baseline in poor quality ECGs where the complexes are not clear or the baseline 'wanders' because of artefact. In this situation, we would advise that the ECG be repeated.

Once you have established whether the ST segment is elevated above or depressed below the isoelectric baseline, the next step is to measure the *amount* of ST segment deviation. For this, you need to identify the so-called *J point*.

J point

The J point is where the QRS complex meets the ST segment (Figure 11.2). ST segment changes should be measured two small squares (i.e. 80 ms) beyond the J point (Figure 11.3). The amount of ST segment deviation (elevation or depression) should be measured in millimetres above or below the isoelectric baseline.

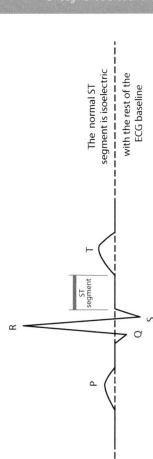

Figure 11.1 The ST segment. Normally, the ST segment is 'isoelectric' with the baseline of the ECG.

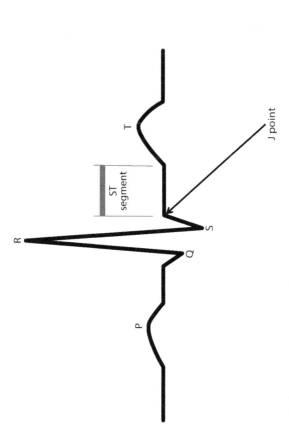

Figure 11.2 The J point. The J point is the point where the QRS complex meets the ST segment.

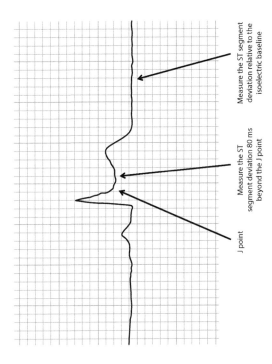

Measure the ST segment deviation relative to the isoelectric baseline

Measure the ST segment deviation 80 ms beyond the J point

J point

Figure 11.3 Measurement of ST segment deviation. ST segment elevation or depression is measured relative to the isoelectric baseline 80 ms after the J point. Here there is 2 mm of ST segment elevation.

ST segment elevation

ST segment elevation is considered significant if there is more than 1 mm elevation two small squares (80 ms) from the J point. The differential diagnosis of ST segment elevation includes the following possibilities:

- ST segment elevation myocardial infarction (STEMI)
- Left ventricular aneurysm
- Prinzmetal's (vasospastic) angina
- Pericarditis
- Early repolarization

ST segment elevation is also a feature of Brugada syndrome (see 'Brugada syndrome' box in Chapter 8).

ST segment elevation myocardial infarction

Commonly, patients suffering from an acute coronary syndrome (ACS) present with a sensation of pressure or tightness at the front of their chest. This may be accompanied by shortness of breath, clamminess, nausea and/or vomiting. Some patients, especially the elderly and those with diabetes, may have minimal symptoms and commonly present primarily with breathlessness.

Clinical context is always important in ECG interpretation. In the context of these clinical features to suggest an ACS, a STEMI is diagnosed when there is

- ≥1 mm of ST segment elevation in two or more contiguous limb leads

Or

- ≥2 mm of ST segment elevation in two or more

CONTIGUOUS LEADS

What does the expression 'contiguous leads' mean?
Contiguous leads means that the leads are next to each other in the *anatomical* sense.

For the limb leads
- The three inferior leads (II, III, aVF) are contiguous
- The two lateral leads (I, aVL) are contiguous

For the chest leads
- Any two of the six leads that are next to each other (e.g. V1 and V2, V2 and V3, etc.) are contiguous

ST segment elevation can be present in more than two leads, but at least two leads must be contiguous for a STEMI to be diagnosed.

We can also use the location of the ST segment elevation in different leads to determine which part(s) of the heart have been affected by myocardial infarction (Table 11.1). Thus, when we refer to an inferior STEMI, this is indicated by ST segment elevation in at least two of the inferior leads (II, III and aVF), and this is usually due to an occlusion of the right coronary artery. An example of an inferior STEMI is shown in Figure 11.4.

Table 11.1 ECG leads and the myocardial territories they correspond to

I	Lateral	aVR	Left main stem	V1	Septal	V4	Anterior
II	Inferior	aVL	Lateral	V2	Septal	V5	Lateral
III	Inferior	aVF	Inferior	V3	Anterior	V6	Lateral

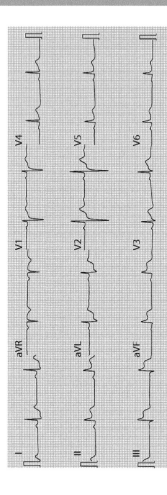

Figure 11.4 Inferior STEMI. There is ST segment elevation in leads II, III and aVF, with 'reciprocal' T segment depression leads I and aVL.

Conversely, a lateral STEMI is indicated by ST segment elevation in at least two of the lateral leads (V5, V6, I and aVL), and is usually due to an occlusion of the circumflex coronary artery. An occlusion of the left anterior descending coronary artery usually causes an anterior ± septal STEMI (Figure 11.5).

Patients with ST segment elevation and symptoms consistent with ACS should have immediate senior review and be considered for *urgent* coronary revascularization, known as primary percutaneous coronary intervention. Any delay, even in minutes, will lead to more of the heart muscle being damaged and increases the risk of permanent disability due to heart failure and death.

ST SEGMENT ELEVATION IN LEAD AVR

Recently, increasing emphasis has been placed on early coronary intervention in 'high-risk' acute coronary syndromes. One particular high-risk variant is left main stem occlusion. The left main stem divides into the left anterior descending and circumflex coronary arteries, and therefore supplies the majority of the left ventricle. If the left main stem becomes occluded, there is a very high risk of substantial damage to the left ventricle, leading to cardiogenic shock and death. In the context of symptoms indicative of ACS plus widespread ST segment depression, the presence of ST segment elevation in lead aVR is suggestive of occlusion of the left main stem and, if ST segment elevation of 1 mm or more is present, predicts a six fold to sevenfold increase in mortality.

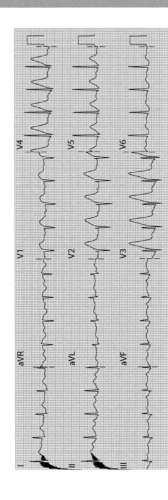

Figure 11.5 Anteroseptal STEMI. There is ST segment elevation in leads V1–V4.

USING ADDITIONAL ELECTRODE POSITIONS

Although the standard 12-lead ECG gives a good overview of the heart, it does not show some areas particularly well. For instance, the posterior aspect of the left ventricle is not well 'seen' properly, nor is the right ventricle. For this reason, it can be helpful to use some additional electrode positions to diagnose the location of posterior or right ventricular STEMIs. The diagnosis of a posterior STEMI is made clearer with the use of posterior leads V7, V8 and V9 (see 'ST segment depression' section). The identification of right ventricular involvement in an inferior STEMI is aided by the use of right-sided chest leads (V1R–V6R), as explained in Chapter 3.

Left ventricular aneurysm

The development of a left ventricular aneurysm is a late complication of myocardial infarction, seen (to varying degrees) in about 10% of survivors. The presence of an aneurysm can lead to persistent ST segment elevation in those chest leads that 'look at' the affected region (Figure 11.6).

If a patient has persistent ST segment elevation due to a left ventricular aneurysm, it is helpful to give them a copy of their ECG to carry. If they present with chest pain in the future, having a copy of an old ECG instantly available for comparison can make it considerably easier to decide whether any ST segment elevation is acute or

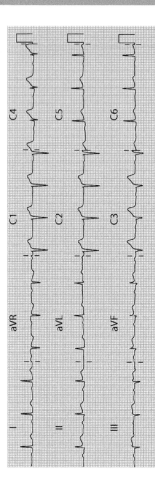

Figure 11.6 Left ventricular aneurysm. Persistent ST segment elevation in leads V1–V4 six months following an anterior STEMI.

Prinzmetal's (vasospastic) angina

Prinzmetal's angina refers to reversible myocardial ischaemia that results from coronary artery spasm. Although any artery can be affected, spasm most commonly occurs in the right coronary artery. During an episode of vasospasm, the patient develops ST segment elevation in the affected territory (Figure 11.7).

Although the combination of chest pain and ST segment elevation often suggests STEMI, vasospastic angina is distinguished by the *transient* nature of the ST segment elevation. Unlike STEMI, the ECG changes of vasospastic angina resolve entirely when the episode of chest pain settles. Episodes of chest pain due to spasm typically occur at rest and particularly overnight. Patients may also have a history of other vasospastic disorders, such as Raynaud's phenomenon.

Pericarditis

The most common non-ischaemic cause of ST segment elevation is pericarditis (inflammation of the lining that surrounds the heart). Clinically, the pain of pericarditis can usually be distinguished from that of myocardial infarction. Although both produce a retrosternal pain, the pain of pericarditis is sharp and pleuritic, exacerbated by inspiration and relieved by sitting forwards.

The ST segment elevation of pericarditis (Figure 11.8) has four characteristics that help to distinguish it from STEMI:

1. The ST segment elevation is typically widespread, affecting all of those leads (anterolateral and inferior) that 'look at' the inflamed epicardium. Leads aVR and V1 usually show reciprocal ST segment depression.

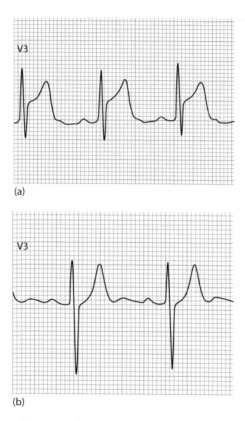

Figure 11.7 Prinzmetal's (vasospastic) angina. ECG shows
(a) anterior ST segment elevation during episode of chest pain and
(b) the ST segment elevation resolving as the chest pain settles.

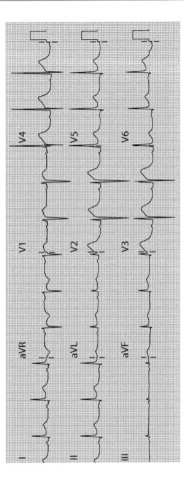

Figure 11.8 Pericarditis. Widespread 'saddle-shaped' ST segment elevation.

2. The ST segment elevation is characteristically 'saddle shaped' (concave upwards).

3. T wave inversion occurs only after the ST segments have returned to baseline.

4. Q waves do not develop.

Pericarditis can also cause depression of the PR segment, which is thought to be caused by atrial involvement in the inflammatory process. PR segment depression is a specific ECG feature of pericarditis and can be very subtle (0.25–0.5 mm). It may be seen in any leads except aVR and V1 (where there may be PR segment elevation).

Early repolarization

Early repolarization, sometimes called 'high take-off', refers to ST segment changes that are non-pathological in nature and are more common in young men. It is important to be aware of early repolarization changes (early repolarization being strictly a term used to describe the observed changes, as the changes have little to do with the process of early repolarization) as they can easily be misinterpreted for ST elevation associated with a heart attack.

Characteristics of early repolarization are

- An upward concave elevation of the ST segment
- Slurring or notching at the J point
- Absence of reciprocal ST segment depression
- Large symmetrical T waves
- Persistence of these changes for many years

ST segment depression

The differential diagnosis of ST segment depression includes the following possibilities:

- Myocardial ischaemia
- Acute posterior myocardial infarction
- Digoxin effect
- Left ventricular hypertrophy with 'strain'

Myocardial ischaemia

During episodes of myocardial ischaemia (angina), patients may develop transient ST segment depression that resolves when the patient rests or uses glyceryl trinitrate (Figure 11.9). More persistent ST elevation that does not resolve shortly after physical exertion or that comes on at rest may be a sign of unstable angina or, if there is a subsequent rise in serum troponin levels, a non-STEMI).

Patients who present with symptoms of ACS plus ST segment depression require urgent senior review with a view to coronary angiography ± coronary reperfusion within 72 h (or more urgently if the patient has ischaemia on the ECG accompanied by ongoing chest pain or hypotension).

Acute posterior myocardial infarction

Approximately 3% of heart attacks will be as a result of a myocardial infarction that primarily affects the posterior wall of the left ventricle, normally due to occlusion of the circumflex coronary artery. Although this is an STEMI, the

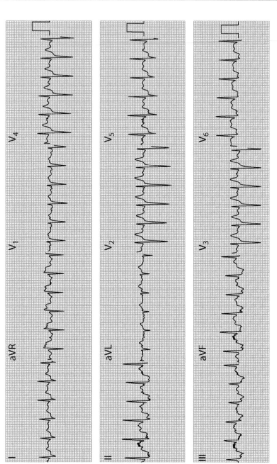

Figure 11.9 Myocardial ischaemia. There is inferolateral ST segment depression.

standard 12-lead ECG will show an ST segment *depression* in the anteroseptal leads V1–V3 (Figure 11.10), accompanied by a large 'dominant' R wave. This is however a reciprocal (mirror image) view of what is happening posteriorly. By performing an ECG using posterior leads (V7, V8 and V9 – see 'Posterior chest leads' section in Chapter 3) the posterior ST segment elevation becomes clear.

Digoxin effect

Digoxin has a characteristic effect on the ST segment, causing an ST segment depression which is described as a 'reverse tick' (Figure 11.11). There may also be T wave inversion. Always distinguish between digoxin *effect*, which may be apparent at therapeutic doses, and digoxin *toxicity*, which indicates overdosage. ST segment depression is seen with normal doses of digoxin and does not in itself indicate overdosage.

Left ventricular hypertrophy with 'strain'

The ECG appearances of left ventricular hypertrophy were discussed in Chapter 10. The 'strain' pattern is said to be present when, in addition to tall R waves and deep S waves, there is also ST segment depression (Figure 10.5). The term 'strain' is rather misleading, because the underlying mechanism is unclear.

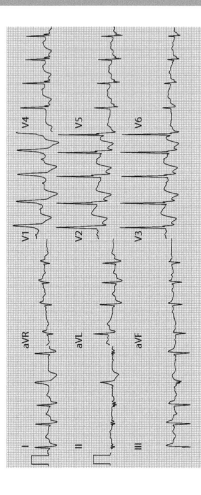

Figure 11.10 Posterior myocardial infarction. There is a dominant R wave in lead V1, with an T segment depression in the anteroseptal chest leads.

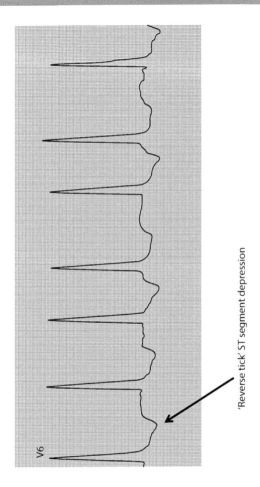

'Reverse tick' ST segment depression

Figure 11.11 Digoxin effect. There is atrial fibrillation and 'reverse tick' ST segment depression.

Further reading

NICE guideline on chest pain of recent onset. (2010). Available at https://www.nice.org.uk/guidance/cg95, accessed 4 August 2015.

NICE guideline on unstable angina and NSTEMI. (2010). Available at https://www.nice.org.uk/guidance/cg94, accessed 4 August 2015.

Marinella MA. Electrocardiographic manifestations and differential diagnosis of acute pericarditis. *Am Fam Physician* 1998; **57**: 699–704.

Wagner GS, Macfarlane P, Wellens H et al. AHA/ACCF/HRS recommendations for the standardization and interpretation of the electrocardiogram: Part VI: Acute ischaemia/infarction. *J Am Coll Cardiol* 2009; **53**: 1003–1011.

T wave changes

The T wave represents the repolarization (recovery) of the ventricles after they have depolarized (Figure 2.5). The T wave is normally upright in all leads except leads V1 and aVR (Figure 12.1). In some cases, T wave inversion can also be normal in lead III.

Tall upright T waves

There is no clearly defined normal range for T wave height, although, as a general rule, a T wave should be no more than half the size of the preceding QRS complex. T waves are usually <5 mm tall in the limb leads, and <15 mm tall in the chest leads. Unusually tall T waves occur in hyperkalaemia and are sometimes an early finding in ST segment elevation myocardial infarction (STEMI).

Hyperkalaemia

Tall and narrow (peaked or 'tented') T waves can indicate high serum potassium levels (Figure 12.2). Hyperkalaemia

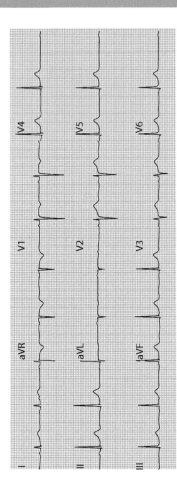

Figure 12.1 Normal 12-lead ECG. The shape and orientation of normal T waves varies from lead to lead.

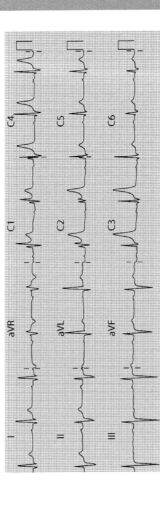

Figure 12.2 Hyperkalaemia. Tall 'tented' T waves are present in the anteroseptal chest leads.

segment is incorporated into the upstroke of the T wave.
Hyperkalaemia may also cause:

- Flattening and even loss of the P wave
- Lengthening of the PR interval
- Shortening of the QT interval
- Widening of the QRS complex, ultimately resembling a
  sine wave
- Arrhythmias (ventricular fibrillation or asystole)

STEMI

Tall narrow T waves can be one of the earliest ECG
features of an acute myocardial infarction (prior to
the patient developing ST segment elevation), and
this possibility should be borne in mind in a patient
presenting with chest discomfort indicative of an ACS.
Such T waves are often referred to as 'hyperacute'
(Figure 12.3).

Small T waves

Just as hyperkalaemia causes tall T waves, so
hypokalaemia causes small T waves (Figure 12.4).
Look carefully for other ECG changes that may
accompany hypokalaemia:

- First-degree heart block
- Depression of the ST segment
- Prominent U waves.

Small T waves can also be a feature of
hypothyroidism (along with small QRS complexes and
sinus bradycardia)

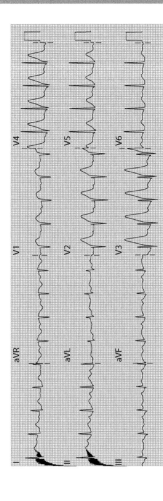

Figure 12.3 Acute anterior myocardial infarction. Tall 'hyperacute' T waves are present in the anteroseptal chest leads.

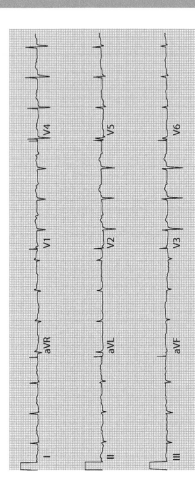

Figure 12.4 Hypokalaemia. There are small T waves and prominent U waves, plus first-degree atrioventricular block and left axis deviation.

Inverted T waves

T wave inversion is considered normal in:
- Leads aVR and V1 (see Figure 12.1)
- Lead V2 in younger people
- Lead V3 in black people

T wave inversion in lead III can also be normal, and may be accompanied by a small Q wave – both of these findings can disappear if the ECG is repeated with the patient's breath held in deep inspiration.

T wave inversion in any other lead is generally considered abnormal, and if it is present, consider whether your patient has one of the following:
- Myocardial ischaemia
- Myocardial infarction
- Ventricular hypertrophy with 'strain' (see Chapter 11)
- Digoxin effect (see Chapter 11)

Myocardial ischaemia

ST segment depression is the commonest manifestation of myocardial ischaemia (Chapter 11), but T wave inversion may also occur in the leads that 'look at' the affected areas. Because ischaemia is reversible, these ECG abnormalities will only be observed during an ischaemic episode.

A particularly high-risk form of ischaemic T wave inversion is seen in *Wellens' syndrome*. This is characterized by symmetrical, deep (>2 mm) T wave inversion in the anterior chest leads (Figure 12.5), often with accompanying horizontal ST segment depression, and is an indicator of impending occlusion of the left anterior descending

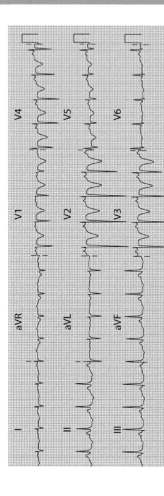

Figure 12.5 Wellens' syndrome. Deep T wave inversion in the anterior chest leads in a patient presenting with unstable angina. Coronary angiography revealed a critical proximal stenosis in the left anterior descending coronary artery.

(LAD) coronary artery. Hence, patients who present with a Wellens' pattern ECG who have (or who have recently had) symptoms of chest pain should have urgent senior review.

Myocardial infarction

T wave inversion can occur not only as a temporary change in myocardial ischaemia but also as a more prolonged change in myocardial infarction. Myocardial infarctions are often divided into (Figure 12.6):

- STEMI
- Non-ST segment elevation myocardial infarction (NSTEMI)

T wave inversion can occur in either type of infarct. T wave inversion may be permanent, or the T wave may return to normal. NSTEMI can also cause T wave inversion, although it can also manifest as ST segment depression alone.

VENTRICULAR ECTOPIC BEATS AND THE T WAVE

Ventricular ectopic beats can be harmless, particularly when the heart is structurally normal, but they can also be a cause of hazardous arrhythmias. Ventricular ectopic beats can occur at the same time as the T wave of the preceding beat – such 'R on T' ventricular ectopic beats (Figure 8.3) can act as a trigger for ventricular tachycardia or fibrillation. Ventricular ectopic beats are discussed in more detail in Chapter 8.

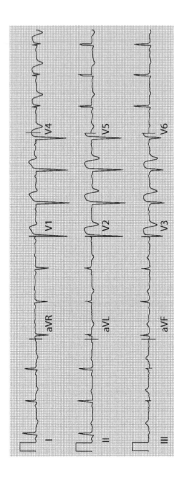

Figure 12.6 Evolving ST segment elevation myocardial infarction. As the ST segment elevation returns to baseline, T wave inversion develops. Note also the development of Q waves in the anterior leads.

Further reading

Mead NE, O'Keefe KP. Wellens' syndrome: An ominous EKG pattern. *J Emerg Trauma Shock* 2009; **2**: 206–208.

Montague BT, Ouellette JR, Buller GK. Retrospective review of the frequency of ECG changes in hyperkalemia. *Clin J Am Soc Nephrol* 2008; **3**: 324–330.

Chapter 13

QT interval prolongation

Many nurses and clinicians have either not been taught the significance of measuring the QT interval or find it difficult. Hence, it is not always given the clinical prominence that it deserves in everyday clinical practice. In this chapter, we explain what the QT interval is and why it matters clinically, and describe some simple ways to measure it.

What is the QT interval?

To put it simply, the QT interval is the time it takes the ventricles of the heart to depolarize and then repolarize again. The ventricles rely on four key salts (sodium, potassium, magnesium and calcium) to generate their electrical current. The movement of these salts into and out of the cells generates the current that we measure and that the heart needs to function.

Prolongation of the repolarization period can make the heart prone to life-threatening ventricular arrhythmias that we will discuss later in this chapter. The longer the period is, the higher the risk that a serious arrhythmia might occur.

Measuring the QT interval

We measure the QT interval from the start of the QRS complex (the start of ventricular depolarization) to the end of the T wave (the end of ventricular repolarization), as shown in Figure 13.1. The measurement of the QT interval can be tricky as we have to decide where the QRS complex starts and where the T wave ends.

THE IMPORTANCE OF U WAVES

U waves (a positive deflection after the T wave) are present on some ECGs, and it is sometimes possible to mistake a U wave for a T wave. This can lead to over-estimation of the QT interval. Therefore always be careful when measuring the QT interval when U waves are present. In this situation, it can be easier to measure the QT interval in leads aVR or aVL, where U waves are usually least prominent.

The QT interval is normally measured in lead II or in leads V5 or V6 (its duration can vary subtly between leads – we should usually measure the QT interval where it is longest). It is important that when we measure the QT interval on different occasions, we should use the same lead for consistency (and so we should record which lead was used for future reference).

When measuring the QT interval manually, the 'maximum slope intercept method' is best:

1. Use lead II (alternatively lead V5 or V6 if lead II is of poor quality).
2. Draw a line through the baseline (preferably the

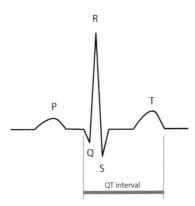

Figure 13.1 **The QT interval.**

3. Draw a tangent against the steepest part of the end of the T wave. If the T wave has two positive deflections, the taller deflection should be chosen. If the T wave is biphasic, the end of the taller deflection should be chosen.

The QT interval starts at the beginning of the QRS complex and ends where the tangent and baseline cross (Figure 13.2). If the QRS duration exceeds 120 ms (such as in a bundle branch block), the amount by which the QRS duration surpasses 120 ms should be deducted from the measured QT interval:

Actual QT interval = Measured QT interval
(QRS duration 120 ms)

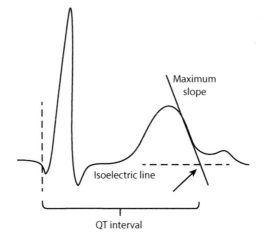

Figure 13.2 **Measurement of the QT interval.**

'Correcting' the QT interval

When assessing the QT interval, it must be corrected for heart rate. The faster the heart rate the shorter the QT interval, and the slower the heart rate the longer the QT interval. Thus, without correction, results cannot be compared.

A QT interval that has been corrected for heart rate is referred to as the *QTc interval* (or 'corrected QT interval'). This is the measurement we should use when comparing ECGs.

Most modern ECG machines can automatically work out the QTc for us (but this function is not always enabled). If your local machine does not display this function, then either consult the manufacturer or your local medical electronics department to get it enabled.

There are many formulas for working out the QTc using different mathematical techniques. If using an ECG machine, it is important to know which formula the machine uses, as different formulas will give slightly different results and cannot be compared like for like. Sometimes the formula used is indicated by an additional letter after QTc, such as QTcB for Bazett's formula or QTcF for Fridericia's formula.

Bazett's formula:

$$QTcB = \frac{QT}{\sqrt{RR}}$$

Fridericia's formula:

$$QTcF = \frac{QT}{\sqrt[3]{RR}}$$

For both these examples, the RR interval must be measured in seconds. As an example, consider a measured QT interval of 400 ms. At a heart rate of 70 beats/min, the RR interval (the time between successive R waves) is 0.86 s. Using these two formulas

Bazett's formula:

$$QTcB = \frac{QT}{\sqrt{RR}} = \frac{400}{\sqrt{0.86}} = 431 \text{ ms}$$

Fridericia's formula:

$$QTcF = \frac{QT}{\sqrt[3]{RR}} = \frac{400}{\sqrt[3]{0.86}} = 421 \text{ ms}$$

As you can see, these two formulas give similar (but slightly different) results for the QTc interval. Bazett's formula is probably the most widely used one in Europe but becomes less accurate at heart rates <60 beats/min and >100 beats/min, so an alternative formula (such as Fridericia's) should be used when bradycardia or tachycardia is present.

A less commonly used formula, that is easier to work out without a calculator, is Hodges formula:

$$QTcH = QT + 1.75 \times (\text{Heart rate} - 60)$$

Applying Hodges formula to the example:

$$
\begin{aligned}
QTcH &= QT + 1.75 \times (\text{Heart rate} - 60) \\
&= 400 + 1.75 \times (70 - 60) \\
&= 400 + 1.75 \times 10 \\
&= 400 + 17.5 \\
&= 417.5 \text{ ms}
\end{aligned}
$$

Alternatively, there are many smartphone apps that you can download that will calculate QTc for you and remove the risk of mathematical error.

THE 'EYEBALL' APPROACH TO QT INTERVAL ASSESSMENT

Probably the most important thing for any nurse to remember when assessing the QT interval is whether the QTc *looks* long, that is the 'eyeball' approach. If it does then check the figures. But what is long? Well, *if the QT interval is longer than half of the RR interval then it may be prolonged* (Figure 13.3), and so an accurate measurement and correction should be performed.

What is a normal QTc interval?

The normal upper limit of QTc differs according to gender:
• For men, the QTc should be less than 450 ms
• For women, the QTc should be less than 460 ms
Anything above these parameters is called a long QT interval. You will see slightly different figures in different textbooks, and this is because the upper limit of QT interval is not a strict 'all or none' cutoff. Rather, the risk of arrhythmias steadily increases the longer the QT interval becomes. Although mildly prolonged QT intervals should not be ignored, the main concern occurs once the QT interval exceeds 500 ms.

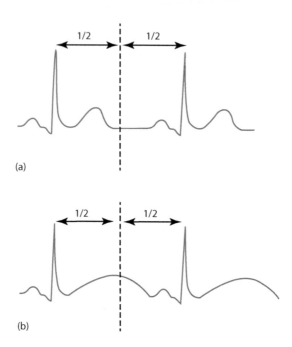

Figure 13.3 The 'eyeball' method of assessing the QT interval. (a) A normal QT interval is usually less than half the RR interval. (b) A prolonged QT interval will be more than half the RR interval.

CAN YOU HAVE A SHORT QT INTERVAL?

It is possible to have a *short* QT interval – the normal lower limit is generally quoted as 360 ms (but different textbooks vary). A short QT interval is extremely rare, but is seen in short QT syndrome. This is an ion channel problem that predisposes to both atrial and ventricular fibrillation, and can present with sudden cardiac death. Short QT syndrome usually requires implantation of an implantable cardioverter-defibrillator (ICD).

Risks of a long QT interval

If the QT interval is prolonged, then the individual is at risk of potentially life-threatening ventricular arrhythmias. The most common of these arrhythmias is a broad complex tachycardia known as *torsades de pointes* (TdP), which translates as 'twisting of the points'. This describes the characteristic appearance on the ECG where there is a continuously varying QRS complex morphology in which the axis constantly changes (Figure 13.4).

TdP is a specific form of polymorphic ventricular tachycardia (VT) occurring in the context of QT prolongation: for TdP to be diagnosed, the patient has to have evidence of polymorphic VT *and* an underlying QT prolongation. TdP runs a risk of precipitating ventricular fibrillation, and so patients can present with cardiac arrest/ sudden cardiac death.

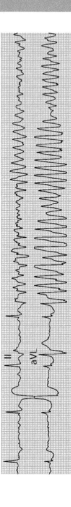

Figure 13.4 Polymorphic ventricular tachycardia (torsades de pointes) triggered by an 'R on T' ventricular ectopic beat.

Causes of a long QT interval

Prolongation of the QT interval can be either inherited or acquired. There are several inherited conditions that prolong the QT interval collectively known as the long QT syndromes (LQTS). These are 'ion channelopathies', caused by a genetic abnormality that affects the function of the cardiac potassium, sodium or calcium ion channels. Several subtypes of LQTS are now described, caused by a variety of different gene mutations. Some of the syndromes also carry the names of those who first described them, such as Romano–Ward syndrome and Jervell and Lange-Nielsen syndrome. The vast majority of cases of LQTS are caused by problems with the potassium channel (LQTS 1 and LQTS 2) or sodium channel (LQTS 3).

Acquired LQTS is normally associated with medication, for example antidepressants. A list of common examples is shown in Table 13.1. The prescribing or administration of drugs that prolong the QT interval should be avoided in patients who are known to have an inherited LQTS. Almost anyone who takes a QT prolonging drug has some risk. Usually, the risk is very low. However, certain risk factors are recognized, including:

- Females
- Structural heart disease
- Electrolyte abnormalities
- Bradycardia
- Hypothermia

Individuals who take more than one drug known to prolong the QT interval, or those who take a combination of drugs (drug–drug interactions) that may cause high blood levels

Table 13.1 Common examples of drugs that can prolong the QT interval

Antiarrhythmics	Amiodarone Dronedarone Flecainide Sotalol
Antibiotics	Erythromycin Clarithromycin Fluconazole
Antidepressants	Amitriptyline Citalopram/escitalopram Haloperidol
Antipsychotics	Chlorpromazine Haloperidol
Antiemetics	Domperidone Ondansetron
Others	Methadone Propofol

of the QT-prolonging drug, are also at particular risk. Individuals who have taken an overdose of a drug known to prolong the QT interval also have increased risk. The nurse should be aware of all the properties of any drug that they prescribe or administer, and if there is any concern, then regular QTc monitoring is advised.

Other conditions that may prolong the QT interval are

- Hypocalcaemia
- Hypokalaemia

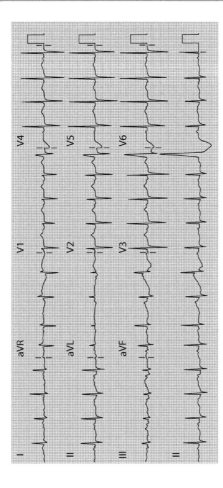

igure 13.5 Prolonged QT interval in an elderly patient with hypocalcaemia.

- Hypothermia
- Myocardial ischemia
- Acute myocarditis
- Raised intracranial pressure (e.g. subarachnoid haemorrhage)

Figure 13.5 shows a 12-lead ECG recorded in an elderly patient with hypocalcaemia and a markedly prolonged QT interval.

Treatment of a long QT interval

Where a treatable underlying cause can be identified (e.g. electrolytes abnormalities or drug treatment), this should be corrected. In hereditary LQTS, careful risk assessment is required to determine the danger of ventricular arrhythmias. Drug treatment (such as beta-blockers) may be appropriate, and an implantable cardioverter-defibrillator (ICD) should be considered in those with a significant risk of sudden cardiac death.

Further reading

Roden DM. Long-QT syndrome. *New Engl J Med* 2008; **358**: 169–176.

van Noord C, Eijgelsheim M, Stricker BHCh. Drug- and non-drug-associated QT interval prolongation. *Br J Clin Pharmacol* 2010; **70**: 16–23.

Chapter 14

Bedside and ambulatory monitoring

In the previous chapters, we focused on 12-lead ECG monitoring. However, a key disadvantage of the traditional 12-lead ECG is that it only takes a 'snapshot' of the heart rhythm over a period of 10 s. If a patient has episodic symptoms that do not occur during that brief period of recording, a significant abnormality can be missed. To get around this problem, there are various modalities that provide for continuous recording over an extended period of time.

Inpatient ECG monitoring

Traditionally, continuous 'bedside' ECG monitoring in hospital is carried out using a three-electrode ECG with electrodes placed on the right arm, left arm and left leg. However, this has two key disadvantages:

1. Most monitors require the patient to be attached to a fixed point (the monitor) and thus reduce the patient's independence/mobility.

This disadvantage can be alleviated by using a 'telemetry' system that utilizes a wireless network to allow the patient some independence while being observed.

2. Three-electrode monitoring systems only provides a limited 'view' of the heart. Hence, while they are excellent for the identification of arrhythmias, they are of little use in monitoring patients with ischaemic symptoms where the nurse is monitoring for possible ST segment changes. This is best undertaken using a 10-electrode (12-lead) monitoring system that gives the same set of 'views' as a traditional 12-lead ECG.

Continuous 10-electrode monitoring is normally undertaken within coronary care units on patients admitted with high-risk acute coronary syndromes or following percutaneous coronary intervention. When performing 10-electrode monitoring, it is common practice to place the limb electrodes on bony prominences (shoulders and iliac crests) to reduce movement artefact – by placing the electrodes over bone instead of muscle, the electrodes are less likely to pick up the electrical activity of muscular contraction. The nurse needs to be aware that ECGs recorded in this way may have subtle changes in QRS axis compared to an ECG recorded in the traditional electrode positions.

MONITORING WITH 5-ELECTRODE SYSTEMS

There are five-electrode monitoring solutions on the market that give a '12-lead view' of the heart (the computer software uses an algorithm to 'estimate' the views that would have been provided by the 'missing' electrodes). These systems have a perceived benefit that they burden the patient with fewer electrodes. However, studies have shown a lack of correlation between what the computer believes is happening and that observed on a traditional 12-lead ECG, and so regulatory bodies have issued caution notices that such systems should not be used to make a diagnosis of acute ischaemia.

One important note for all nurses using continuous monitoring is to be aware of the 'clinical alarm fatigue syndrome'. This is a well documented process where the nurse does not set the triggers for patient alarms appropriately. This can lead to frequent inappropriate alarms that ultimately result in the desensitization of the nurse to 'genuine' alarms. Hence, the response to a genuine alarm can end up being delayed. Regular alarm noise is also often cited by patients as affecting their sleep and promoting anxiety in critical care units, and so should be avoided.

Outpatient ECG monitoring

Heart rhythm problems or palpitations (awareness of the heart beating) are experienced by more than a million people a year in the United Kingdom and are in the top

10 reasons why people attend hospital. There are several outpatient monitoring options available depending on the frequency at which symptoms occur.

Continuous ambulatory monitors

By far, the most common form of ambulatory ECG monitoring is the 24-hour ambulatory ECG (often referred to as a Holter monitor or '24-hour tape'). This consists of a three-electrode ECG connected to a mobile monitor that the patient wears in a holster.

It is important to be aware of the limitations of 24-hour ambulatory ECG monitoring. The specificity of these devices have been cited as being as high as 96.6%. However, the sensitivity can be as low as 2%. Simply put, they are very good at identifying an arrhythmia if you happen to have it whilst you are wearing the device, but not so good at ruling out an arrhythmia if you happen to be asymptomatic while wearing the device.

Hence, a 'negative' result can be falsely reassuring. If a patient did not have his or her usual symptoms while wearing the monitor, then we may simply have not had a chance to capture an arrhythmia. The length of time that an ambulatory ECG monitor is worn can be extended to several days but, pragmatically, if you ask a patient to wear a monitor for more than 48 h then patient acceptance declines as it gets uncomfortable to wear and they cannot easily shower or bathe.

Cardiomemo devices

When patients experience infrequent symptoms, then

ECG during a symptomatic event. One technique is to give the patient a two-electrode device to record an ECG 'on demand'. This is often referred to as a 'cardiomemo' device.

The patient carries one of these devices with them and, when they experience their usual symptoms, they hold the device to their chest and record an ECG. Whilst getting around the problem of having to wear a monitor for days on end, this type of device is prone to movement artefact and is also no good for screening for asymptomatic arrhythmias or for capturing the rhythm during an episode of transient loss of consciousness (TLoC).

Implantable ECG loop recorders

For patients with a suspected cardiac arrhythmic cause of TLoC, occurring less than once every 2 weeks, the National Institute for Health and Care Excellence suggests that the clinician should offer implantation of a cardiac rhythm monitoring device known as an implantable loop recorder (ILR, Figure 14.1). This offers the most effective way to try and capture the ECG during an episode of TLoC.

Apart from being used in TLoC, these implantable devices have a role to play in ruling out atrial fibrillation (AF) in cryptogenic stroke (stroke of no known cause). Evidence suggests that 15% of all strokes, and up to 40% of cryptogenic strokes, are secondary to asymptomatic episodes of AF. One recent study suggested that 30% of patients who had an ILR implanted were found to have significant episodes of AF detected within 3 years of their cryptogenic

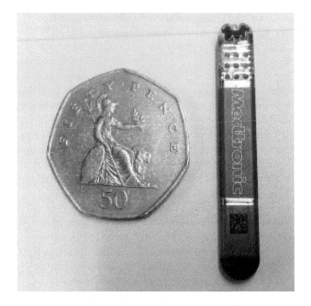

Figure 14.1 An implantable ECG loop recorder (Medtronic Reveal LINQ device) with a 50 pence coin for scale.

The newer type of ILRs are 'injected' under the skin over the chest wall under local anaesthetic in a procedure that takes approximately 15 min. The wound is closed with either Steri-Strips or surgical glue. Patient acceptance is high and surgical trauma and scarring minimalized. These devices are designed for the clinic setting and do not require the patient to go to a theatre or a cardiac catheter

These newer devices also utilize remote monitoring technology (mobile phone networks) that allow the patient's ECG recordings to be monitored from home, removing the need for the patient to attend hospital if they experience a symptom.

The future of ECG monitoring

ECG applications for iOS and Android smartphones are already available that allow cardiac rhythms to be recorded. At present, these apps require a plug-in interface that either utilizes a two-electrode ECG monitor built into a removable smartphone case or that allows two wired electrodes to be attached to the person. These devices are inexpensive and are freely available online. Hence, in the very near future, patients will attend the emergency department or outpatient clinic with a smartphone and say 'I've recorded my palpitation, and here it is…'.

What does the future hold for monitoring patients in hospital? As technology develops and costs reduce, the traditional cardiac monitor will become a thing of the past (as will the blood pressure monitor). Increasingly, people are turning towards 'wearable' technology as the norm, for example the Apple Watch.

There are already companies that offer wearable devices to monitor heart rate and blood pressure for outpatient investigation. The next generation of such devices will be in the form of a watch or patch that continuously monitors the patient's heart rate/rhythm/temperature/blood pressure and communicates directly with the hospital IT systems, for electronic prescribing and administration. Patients will have their observations continuously recorded with the data uploaded to the hospital's data network on a minute-by-minute basis. Before long, nursing observation rounds will be consigned to history...

Further reading

Graham KC, Cvach M. Monitor alarm fatigue: standardizing use of physiological monitors and decreasing nuisance alarms. *Am J Critical Care* 2010; **19**: 28–35.

NICE guideline on transient loss of consciousness in adults and young people. (2010). Available at https://www.nice.org.uk/guidance/cg109, accessed 4 August 2015.

Roebuck A, Mercer C, Denman J, Houghton AR, Andrews R. Experiences from a non-medical, non-catheter laboratory implantable loop recorder (ILR) service. *Br J Cardiol* 2015; **22**: 36–38.

Chapter 15

Summary of key points

This section contains a 'quick reference' summary of the key points from each of the chapters in this book.

Basics of the heartbeat

The heart consists of four chambers:
- Left and right atria
- Left and right ventricles

Contraction of the ventricles is called *systole*. The period in between ventricular contractions is called *diastole*.

The heart is made up of highly specialized cardiac muscle comprising myocardial cells (myocytes). Myocytes are capable of being
- Pacemaker cells
- Conducting cells
- Contractile cells

The brain tells the heart's natural pacemaker how quickly to beat via two branches of the autonomic nervous system:
1. Sympathetic
2. Parasympathetic

The contraction of the heart chambers and the coordination of its timing are controlled by the heart's electrical system:

- Sinoatrial (SA) node
- Atrioventricular (AV) node
- Bundle of His
- Right and left bundle branches
- Purkinje fibres

Basics of the ECG

A standard 12-lead ECG recording uses 10 electrodes to make a recording that provides 12 'views' of the heart from different angles.

The waves and intervals of the ECG correspond to the following events:

ECG event	Cardiac event
P wave	Atrial depolarization
PR interval	Start of atrial depolarization to start of ventricular depolarization
QRS complex	Ventricular depolarization
ST segment	Pause in ventricular electrical activity before repolarization
T wave	Ventricular repolarization
QT interval	Total time taken by ventricular depolarization and repolarization
U wave	Uncertain – possibly:
	interventricular septal repolarization
	slow ventricular repolarization

> **NB** – Depolarization of the SA and AV nodes are important events but do not in themselves produce a detectable wave on the standard ECG.

A resting *heart rate* of between 60 and 100 beats/min is the normal range for an adult:

- Bradycardia is a heart rate of less than 60 beats/min.
- Tachycardia is a heart rate of greater than 100 beats/min.

The *PR interval* is measured from the beginning of the P wave to the beginning of the QRS complex:

- Short PR interval is <120 ms.
- Normal PR interval is 120–200 ms.
- Long PR interval is >200 ms.

The *QRS duration* is measured from the beginning of the Q wave to the end of the S wave:

- Normal QRS duration is <120 ms.
- Prolonged QRS duration ('broad QRS') is >120 ms.

The *QRS axis* is an indicator of the general direction that the wave of depolarization takes as it flows through the ventricles:

- A normal cardiac axis lies between −30° and +90°.
- Left axis deviation lies between −30° and −90°.
- Right axis deviation lies between +90° and +180°.
- Extreme right axis deviation lies between −90° and −180°.

A QUICK METHOD TO ASSESS THE QRS AXIS

A positive QRS complex in both leads I and II means the *axis is normal.*

A positive QRS complex in lead I and a negative QRS complex in lead II mean there is *left axis deviation.*

A negative QRS complex in lead I and a positive QRS complex in lead II mean there is *right axis deviation.*

A negative QRS complex in lead I and a negative QRS complex in lead II mean there is *extreme right axis deviation.*

How to record a 12-lead ECG

- Explain the procedure to the patient and obtain their consent.
- Ensure the patient is comfortable.
- Prepare the skin before applying the electrodes.
  - Removal of chest hair
  - Light abrasion
  - Skin cleansing
- Place the electrodes correctly.
- Only use ECG filters where necessary, and note this on the ECG.
- Check that the ECG recording is of good quality.
- Label the ECG recording appropriately.
- Ensure that any clinically urgent abnormalities are acted upon.

How to read a 12-lead ECG

To read a 12-lead ECG, review the following features:

- Patient data
  - Patient name
  - Patient gender
  - Date of birth
  - Identification number (e.g. hospital or NHS number)
- Clinical data
  - Reason for the request
  - Relevant past medical history
  - Relevant medication
- Technical data
  - Date and time of recording
  - Paper speed and calibration
  - Technical quality
  - Any non-standard settings
- ECG fundamentals
  - Rate
  - Rhythm
  - Axis
- ECG details
  - P wave
  - PR interval
  - Q wave
  - QRS complex
  - ST segment
  - T wave
  - QT interval

- U wave
- Additional features (e.g. delta wave)

Heart rate: Tachycardia and bradycardia

There are three methods for calculating heart rate in beats/min from the ECG:

1. Count the number of large squares between two consecutive QRS complexes, and divide 300 by that number.
2. Count the number of small squares between two consecutive QRS complexes, and divide 1500 by that number.
3. Count the number of QRS complexes in 50 large squares (the length of the rhythm strip on standard ECG) and multiply by 6.

Bradycardia is a heart rate below 60 beats/min, and common causes to consider are

- Sinus bradycardia
- Sick sinus syndrome
- Second-degree and third-degree AV block
- 'Escape' rhythms
  - AV junctional escape rhythm
  - Ventricular escape rhythms
- Asystole

Tachycardia is a heart rate above 100 beats/min, and common causes to consider are:

- Narrow-complex tachycardias (QRS width <3 small squares):
  - Sinus tachycardia
  - Atrial tachycardia

- Atrial flutter
- Atrial fibrillation
- AV re-entry tachycardia (AVRT)
- AV nodal re-entry tachycardia (AVNRT)
- Broad-complex tachycardias (QRS width >3 small squares):
  - Ventricular tachycardia
  - Accelerated idioventricular rhythm
  - Torsades de pointes
  - A supraventricular tachycardia with aberrant conduction

Approach to heart rhythms

To identify an ECG rhythm, always keep in mind these two key points:

1. Where does the impulse arise from?
   a. Sinoatrial (SA) node
   b. Atria
   c. Atrioventricular (AV) junction
   d. Ventricles
2. How is the impulse conducted?
   a. Normal conduction
   b. Impaired conduction
   c. Accelerated conduction (e.g. Wolff–Parkinson–White syndrome)

To narrow down the diagnostic possibilities, work through the ECG while asking yourself the following seven questions:

1. How is the patient?
2. Is ventricular activity present?

3. What is the ventricular rate?
4. Is the ventricular rhythm regular or irregular?
5. Is the QRS complex width normal or broad?
6. Is atrial activity present?
7. How are atrial activity and ventricular activity related?

Supraventricular rhythms

Supraventricular rhythms are those which originate above the level of the ventricles, that is from the SA node, the atria or the AV node. These include
- Sinus rhythm
- Sinus arrhythmia
- Sinus bradycardia
- Sinus tachycardia
- Sick sinus syndrome
- Atrial ectopic beats
- Atrial fibrillation
- Atrial flutter
- Atrial tachycardia
- AVRT
- AVNRT

Ventricular rhythms

Ventricular rhythms are those which arise from the ventricles, that is below the level of the atrioventricular node. These include
- Ventricular ectopic beats (VEBs)
- Accelerated idioventricular rhythm

- Polymorphic ventricular tachycardia
- Ventricular fibrillation (VF)

Remember that a broad-complex tachycardia can have two possible explanations:

1. The tachycardia may be ventricular in origin (*VT*).
2. The tachycardia may be supraventricular in origin, but have a broad-complex rather than narrow-complex appearance because of a co-existent conduction problem, such as a bundle branch block (*SVT with aberrant conduction*).

THE GOLDEN RULE

A broad-complex tachycardia is always assumed to be VT unless proven otherwise.

Conduction problems and types of block

Problems with cardiac conduction can occur at *four key points*:

1. SA node
   a. SA block
2. AV node (or bundle of His)
   a. First-degree AV block
   b. Second-degree AV block
       i.   Mobitz type I AV block (Wenckebach)
       ii. Mobitz type II AV block
   c. Third-degree AV block
3. Left or right bundle branches
   a. Left bundle branch block (LBBB)

  4. Left anterior or posterior fascicles
     a. Left anterior fascicular block (LAFB)
     b. Left posterior fascicular block (LPFB)

Escape rhythms occur when there is failure of normal impulse generation or conduction, and can arise from the

- AV junction (AV node/bundle of His)
- Ventricular myocardium

QRS complexes and left ventricular hypertrophy

The QRS complex corresponds to ventricular depolarization. Small 'septal' Q waves

- Are normal in leads I, aVL, V5 and V6
- Can be normal in leads III and aVR

Q waves in other leads are 'pathological', if they are

- >2 small squares deep, or
- >25% of the height of the following R wave in depth, and/or
- >1 small square wide

Sokolow–Lyon criteria for left ventricular hypertrophy:

- R wave >11 mm in lead aVL

Or

- Sum of S wave in lead V1 plus the tallest R wave in either lead V5 or V6 >35 mm

Right ventricular hypertrophy may be present if the patient has a normal QRS complex duration and

- Right axis deviation (negative QRS in lead I and positive QRS in lead II)
- R wave in V1 is ≥6 mm in height
- A dominant S wave of ≥6 mm in depth in either V5 or V6

Small QRS complexes may be a variant of normal, or can be due to
- Obesity
- Emphysema
- Pericardial effusion

The normal QRS complex duration is <120 ms.

Broad complexes indicate slow ventricular depolarization due to
- LBBB or RBBB
- Ventricular rhythms (e.g. VEBs, VT, ventricular pacing)

ST segment elevation and depression

The J point is where the QRS complex meets the ST segment (Figure 11.2). ST segment changes should be measured two small squares (i.e. 80 ms) beyond the J point (Figure 11.3).

The differential diagnosis of ST segment elevation includes the following possibilities:
- ST segment elevation myocardial infarction (STEMI)
- Left ventricular aneurysm
- Prinzmetal's (vasospastic) angina
- Pericarditis
- Early repolarization

The differential diagnosis of ST segment depression includes the following possibilities:
- Myocardial ischaemia
- Acute posterior myocardial infarction
- Digoxin effect
- Left ventricular hypertrophy with 'strain'

T wave changes

The T wave represents the repolarization (recovery) of the ventricles after they have depolarized.

T waves should be no more than half the size of the preceding QRS complex. T waves are usually <5 mm tall in the limb leads and <15 mm tall in the chest leads.

Tall T waves can indicate
- Hyperkalaemia
- Early STEMI ('hyperacute T waves')

Small T waves can indicate
- Hypokalaemia
- Hypothyroidism

T wave inversion can indicate
- Myocardial ischaemia
- Myocardial infarction
- Ventricular hypertrophy with 'strain'
- Digoxin effect

QT interval prolongation

The QT interval represents the time taken for ventricular depolarization and repolarization.

The QT interval is measured from the start of the QRS complex to the end of the T wave. As a rule of thumb, the QT interval should usually be less than half the RR interval.

Once measured, the QT interval must be corrected for heart rate to give the corrected QT interval (QTc):
- For men, the QTc should be less than 450 ms.
- For women, the QTc should be less than 460 ms.

Prolongation of the QT interval can result from
- Hereditary long QT syndrome
- Drug effects
- Electrolyte abnormalities

A prolonged QT interval increases the risk of ventricular arrhythmias and can lead to sudden cardiac death.

Treatment options for a long QT interval include
- Removal of any reversible cause
- Drug therapy (e.g. beta-blockers)
- ICD implantation

Short QT syndrome is extremely rare, and is suspected when the QTc is less than 360 ms.

Bedside and ambulatory monitoring

Continuous 'bedside' ECG monitoring in hospital is often carried out using a three-electrode ECG with electrodes placed on the right arm, left arm and left leg.

Continuous 10-electrode monitoring is more cumbersome but allows for a full 12-lead ECG monitoring.

Outpatient ECG monitoring can be undertaken using
- 24-h ambulatory ECG monitors
- Prolonged continuous ambulatory ECG monitoring
- Cardiomemo devices
- Implantable ECG loop recorders

The appropriate duration (and modality) of ECG monitoring should be chosen to maximize the chances of capturing the ECG during a symptomatic event.

Appendix A: ECG resources

Textbooks

Houghton AR, Gray D. *Making Sense of the ECG: A Hands-on Guide*, 4th edn. Boca Raton, FL: CRC Press, 2014. ISBN: 978-1444181821.

Houghton AR. *Making Sense of the ECG: Cases for Self-assessment*, 2nd edn. Boca Raton, FL: CRC Press, 2014. ISBN: 978-1444181845.

Springhouse Publishing. *ECG interpretation Made Incredibly Easy!*, 5th edn. Philadelphia, PA: Lippincott Williams & Wilkins, 2010. ISBN: 978-1608312894.

Key guidelines

Key guidance published by the Society for Cardiological Science and Technology (available from http://www.scst.org.uk, accessed 4 August 2015):

- SCST. *Recording a Standard 12-Lead Electrocardiogram* (2014).
- Macfarlane PW, Coleman EN. *Resting 12-Lead ECG Electrode Placement and Associated Problems* (1995).

Key guidance published by the American College of Cardiology (available from http://www.cardiosource.org, accessed 4 August 2015) in partnership with its sister organizations:

- Recommendations for the Standardization and Interpretation of the Electrocardiogram:

- Kligfield P, Gettes LS, Bailey JJ *et al.* Part 1 – The Electrocardiogram and its Technology *J Am Coll Cardiol.* 2007; **49**: 1109–1127.
- Mason JW, Hancock EW, Gettes LS. Part 2 – Electrocardiography Diagnostic Statement List *J Am Coll Cardiol.* 2007; **49**: 1128–1135.
- Surawicz B, Childers R, Deal BJ *et al.* Part 3 – Intraventricular Conduction Disturbances *J Am Coll Cardiol.* 2009; **53**: 976–981.
- Rautaharju PM, Surawicz B, Gettes LS. Part 4 – The ST Segment, T and U Waves, and the QT Interval *J Am Coll Cardiol.* 2009; **53**: 982–991.
- Hancock EW, Deal BJ, Mirvis DM *et al.* Part 5 – Electrocardiogram Changes Associated with Cardiac Chamber Hypertrophy *J Am Coll Cardiol.* 2009; **53**: 992–1002.
- Wagner GS, Macfarlane P, Wellens H *et al.* Part 6 – Acute Ischaemia/Infarction *J Am Coll Cardiol.* 2009; **53**: 1003–1011.

- Kadish AH, Buxton AE, Kennedy HL *et al.* ACC/AHA Clinical Competence Statement on Electrocardiography and Ambulatory Electrocardiography *J Am Coll Cardiol.* 2001; **38**: 2091–2100.
- Cain ME, Mason JW, Anderson JL *et al.* ACC Expert Consensus Document on Signal-Averaged Electrocardiography *J Am Coll Cardiol.* 1996; **27**: 238–249.

Online learning

The following websites are particularly useful for anyone wanting to learn more about ECG interpretation:

- *ECG pedia*: http://en.ecgpedia.org/wiki/Main_Page, accessed 4 August 2015.
- *ECG Learning Center*: http://ecg.utah.edu, accessed 4 August 2015.
- *Life in the Fast Lane ECG Library*: http://lifeinthefastlane. com/ecg-library/, accessed 4 August 2015.
- *Medmastery*: http://www.medmastery.com/, accessed 4 August 2015.
- *Skillstat ECG Simulator*: http://www.skillstat.com/tools/ ecg-simulator, accessed 4 August 2015.

Societies

Arrhythmia Alliance Website: http://www.heartrhythmcharity. org.uk/, accessed 4 August 2015.

British Heart Rhythm Society Website: http://www.bhrs.com/, accessed 4 August 2015.

European Cardiac Arrhythmia Society Website: http://www. ecas-heartrhythm.org/, accessed 4 August 2015.

Heart Rhythm Society Website: http://www.hrsonline.org/, accessed 4 August 2015.

Appendix B: Help with the next edition

We would like to know what should be included (or omitted!) in the next edition of *Pocket ECGs for Nurses*. Please write with your comments or suggestions to

Dr. Andrew R. Houghton
c/o CRC Press/Taylor & Francis Group
2 Park Square, Milton Park
Abingdon, Oxon OX14 4RN, UK

We will acknowledge all suggestions that are used.

Index

A

ABCDE approach, *see* Airway,
    Breathing, Circulation,
    Disability, Exposure
    (ABCDE) approach
Abnormal cardiac axis, 23
Accelerated idioventricular
    rhythm
    antiarrhythmic drugs, 114
    causes, 111
    occurrence, 111, 113
Accessory pathway, 94, 96
Acute anterior myocardial
    infarction, 190–191
Acute posterior myocardial
    infarction
    J point and, 231
    ST segment depression,
    181, 183
Adrenergic, 6
AF, *see* Atrial fibrillation (AF)
Airway, Breathing, Circulation,
    Disability, Exposure
    (ABCDE) approach
    arrhythmia, 66
    bradycardia, 57–58
    tachycardia, 61
    ventricular rhythms, 116–117
Anteroseptal STEMI, 173–174
Antiarrhythmic drugs

accelerated idioventricular
    rhythm, 114
    QT interval prolongation, 210
    ventricular fibrillation, 127
Antidromic AVRT, 99, 102
Apple Watch, 219
Arrhythmias
    asymptomatic, 217
    diagnosis, 13, 65
    fatal, precipitation, 111
    hyperkalaemia and, 190
    malignant risk, 111
    recognition, 77
    ventricular
        broad-complex tachycardia,
        61, 233
        Brugada syndrome, 118
Arrhythmogenic right ventricular
    cardiomyopathy
    (ARVC), 118
Asymptomatic bifascicular
    block, 145
Asystole
    bradycardia, 54, 56
    heart rhythms, 67–68
    tachycardia, 226
    ventricular, 69, 146
Atrial activity, cardiac rhythm
    atrial depolarization, 74
    categories, 74

fibrillation waves, 75
flutter waves, 75
P waves, 74–75
and ventricular activity, 75–76
Atrial depolarization
atrial electrical activity, 74–75
ECG waves and intervals,
18, 222
Atrial ectopic beats; *see also*
Ventricular ectopic
beats (VEBs)
AVRT in WPW syndrome, 99
supraventricular rhythms,
86–87
Atrial fibrillation (AF)
atrial impulses transmission, 88
chaotic depolarization, 88
chemical cardioversion, 90
low-amplitude oscillations,
88–89
rhythm control, 90–91
stroke risk reduction, 88–90
ventricular rate control, 90
Atrial flutter; *see also* Flutter waves
atrial impulses, 91
impulse looping, 91
management, 91
sawtooth appearance
flutter waves, 91–92
QRS complex initiation,
91, 93
Atrial impulses
atrial flutter, 91

fusion beats, 120
in second-degree AV
block, 54
transmission, 88
Atrial kick, 3
Atrial premature beats
(APBs), 86
Atrial premature complexes
(APCs), 86
Atrial tachycardia
narrow-complex tachycardias,
57, 226
sick sinus syndrome, 86
supraventricular rhythms,
94–95
WPW syndrome, 102
Atrioventricular dissociation,
119–120
Atrioventricular (AV)
node, 18
conducting cells, 6
electrical system, heart, 9
first-degree block
feature, 130, 133
PR interval,
130, 132
problems (*see* Conduction
problems)
second-degree block
Mobitz type I AV block,
133–134
Mobitz type II AV block,
133, 135

third-degree block
  causes, 137
  sinus rhythm, 138
  ventricular escape
    rhythm, 136
Autonomic nervous system, 6, 221
AV nodal re-entry tachycardia
    (AVNRT)
  and AVRT, 105
  micro re-entry circuit, 103
  narrow complex tachycardia,
    104–105
  treatment, 105
AV re-entry tachycardia (AVRT)
  accessory pathway, 94, 96
  antegrade conduction, 96
  antidromic, 99, 102
  delta wave, 96–97
  His–Purkinje system, 97
  orthodromic, 99, 101
  termination, 102–103
  Valsalva manoeuvre, 102–103
  ventricular pre-excitation, 97–98
  WPW pattern
    atrial fibrillation in, 102
    PR interval, 99–100

B

Bazett's formula, QTc interval,
    203–204
Bedside and ambulatory
    monitoring
  ECG applications, 219

clinical alarm fatigue
    syndrome, 215
continuous 10-electrode
    monitoring, 214, 233
disadvantages, 213–214
five-electrode monitoring
    solutions, 215
regular alarm noise, 215
three-electrode ECG,
    213–214
outpatient ECG monitoring
  cardiomemo devices,
    216–217
  continuous ambulatory
    monitors, 216, 233
  heart rhythm problems,
    215–216
  implantable loop recorders
    (see Implantable ECG
    loop recorders)
Bifascicular block, 145
Bradycardia; see also Heart rate
  ABCDE approach, 57–58, 60
  asystole, 54, 56
  causes of
    asystole, 56
    escape rhythms, 56
    second-degree AV block, 54
    sick sinus syndrome, 54
    sinus bradycardia, 54–55
    third-degree AV block, 54
  drug treatment, 56
  negatively chronotropic

resting heart rate, 17
The Resuscitation Council
(UK) 2010 algorithm,
57–58
sick sinus syndrome, 86
ventricular rate, 52
Broad-complex tachycardia, 61,
114–115, 119
Broad QRS complex
causes, 159
left and right bundle branch
blocks, 161
narrow and, 160
Brugada syndrome
monomorphic ventricular
tachycardia, 118
ST segment elevation, 170
Bundle branch block, *see* Left
bundle branch block
(LBBB); Right bundle
branch block (RBBB)
Bundle of His
cells, 6
conduction, 129–130
heart's electrical system,
9, 222

C

Capture beats, 120, 123
Cardiac action potential, 7–8
Cardiac conduction system, 7–8
Cardiac myocytes, 7
Cardiac resynchronization therapy

Cardiac rhythm
ABCDE approach, 66
arrhythmias, 65, 77
atrial activity (*see* Atrial
activity, cardiac
rhythm)
ECG characteristics, 76–77
haemodynamic instability, 67
impulse, 65
patient, 66–67
QRS complex
conduction problems,
72–73
supraventricular rhythm,
73–74
ventricular ectopics, 73
ventricular myocardium, 72
ventricular rhythms, 70, 72
regular and irregular, 70–71
ventricular activity (*see*
Ventricular activity,
cardiac rhythm)
ventricular rate, 69
ventricular rhythm, 69–70
Cardiomemo devices, 216–217, 233
Chaotic depolarization, 88
Chemical cardioversion, 90
Cholinergic, 6
Clinical alarm fatigue
syndrome, 215
Complete heart block, 90, 136
Conducting cells, 6, 221
Conduction blocks,

Conduction problems
AV node
first-degree AV block, 130,
132–133
second-degree AV block
(*see* Second-degree AV
block)
third-degree AV block
(*see* Third-degree
AV block)
escape rhythms, 146–147, 230
fascicular block
(*see* Fascicular block)
LBBB
causes, 139, 141
CRT pacemaker, 139
ECG in, 139–140
interventricular
dyssynchrony, 139
pre-existing, 139, 141
Purkinje fibres, 137
QRS complex
morphology, 120
QRS complex
shapes, 139
Sgarbossa criteria, 141
RBBB
causes, 141–142
ECG features, 120
interventricular
dyssynchrony, 142
interventricular
septum, 144

SA node
atria, 129–130
cardiac conduction, 299
P waves, 130–131
Contiguous leads, 170–171
Continuous ambulatory
monitors, 216
Continuous 10-electrode
monitoring, 214, 233
Contractile cells, 6, 221
Coronary revascularization, 173

D

Delta wave, 96–97, 99–100
Depolarization–repolarization
cycle, 7
Depression, ST segment
acute posterior myocardial
infarction (*see* Acute
posterior myocardial
infarction)
differential diagnosis,
181, 231
digoxin effect, 183, 185
left ventricular hypertrophy
with 'strain,' 183
myocardial ischaemia,
181–182
Dextrocardia
right-sided chest leads, 32–33
12-lead ECG recording, 34
Diastole
definition, 1

Digoxin effect
    ST segment depression, 183,
        185, 231
    T wave inversion, 193, 232
Dyssynchrony
    electrical system anatomy, 7
    interventricular, 139, 142

E

ECG leads
    electrodes, 11
    heart's electrical activity, 11
    limb lead, 13–14
    myocardium, 13
    viewpoints, 11–12
ECG waves
    and cardiac event, 16, 18, 222
    principal, 17–18
    repolarization, 14
    sinoatrial (SA) node, 14
Electrical system, heart
    atrioventricular node, 9
    bundle branches, 10
    bundle of His, 9
    cardiac action potential, 7–8
    cardiac conduction
        system, 7–8
    dyssynchrony, 7
    Purkinje fibres, 10
    sinoatrial node, 9
Electrocardiogram (ECG)
    abnormal cardiac axis, 23
    heart rate, 223

leads (*see* ECG leads)
normal values
    nurses and, 16
    QRS duration, 19
    QT interval, 19
    resting heart rate, 17
    PR interval, 18, 223
    QRS axis (*see* QRS
        (cardiac) axis)
    resources, 235–237
    waves (*see* ECG waves)
Electrode placement, 12-lead ECG
        recording
    chest (precordial) electrodes,
        28, 30–31
    colour codes, 27
    in female patients, 31
    limb electrodes, 28
    misplacement, 28
    parts, 27
    "Ride Your Green Bike", 28
Electrophysiological
        ablation, 111
Elevation, ST segment
    differential diagnosis, 231
    early repolarization, 180
    left ventricular aneurysm,
        175–176
    pericarditis, 177, 179–180
    Prinzmetal's (vasospastic)
        angina, 177–178
    STEMI (*see* ST segment
        elevation myocardial

Escape rhythms
  bradycardia, 54, 56, 226
  cardiac contraction, 6
  conduction problems and block
    types, 146–147, 230
  ventricular, 226
Eyeball approach, QT interval,
  205–206

F

Fascicular block
  asymptomatic bifascicular
    block, 145
  bifascicular block, 145
  conduction blocks,
    combinations, 146
  hemiblock, 144
  LAFB, 144–145
  LPFB, 145
  trifascicular block, 145
Fatal arrhythmias, 111
First-degree AV block, 130, 132–133
Five-electrode monitoring
  solutions, 215
Flutter waves, 74–75, 91
Fridericia's formula, QTc interval,
  203–204
Fusion beats, 120, 122

H

Haemodynamic stability, 119
Heart
  anatomy, 5

atria, 3
atrial kick, 3
diastole, 1, 4
resting heart rate, 3
right ventricle, 3, 5
systole, 1, 4
electric system (see Electrical
  system, heart)
failure, 67
location, 1–2
myocytes, 5–6
vessels, 5
Heart rate
  arrhythmias, 47
  automated calculation, 52
  bradycardia (see Bradycardia)
  large squares counting,
    48–49
  P wave rate, 52
  QRS complexes counting
    automated heart rate
      calculations, 52
    ventricular rate calculation,
      50–51
  small squares counting, 48, 50
  and tachycardia (see
    Tachycardia)
  ventricular rate, 47
Heart rhythms
  cardiac rhythm identification
    (see Cardiac rhythm)
  features, 227–228
  rhythm strip, 63–64

High-risk acute coronary
syndromes, 173
His–Purkinje system
AVRT, 97
broad QRS complexes,
73–74, 159
supraventricular rhythms,
73, 102
ventricular myocardium, 72
ventricular pacing, 161
Hodges formula, QTc interval, 204
Hyperkalaemia
serum potassium levels,
187, 189
T waves, 190, 232
Hypokalaemia
QT interval, 210
T waves, 190, 192
ventricular ectopic beats, 108
Hypothyroidism
sinus bradycardia, 82
third-degree atrioventricular
block, 137
T wave changes, 190, 232

I

Implantable ECG loop recorders
cryptogenic stroke, AF, 217
with 50 pence coin for scale,
217–218
patient acceptance, 218
remote monitoring
technology, 219

Independent P wave activity,
120–121
Inferior myocardial infarction,
151–152
Inpatient ECG monitoring
clinical alarm fatigue
syndrome, 215
continuous 10-electrode
monitoring, 214
disadvantages, 213–214
five-electrode monitoring
solutions, 215
regular alarm noise, 215
three-electrode ECG, 213–214
Interventricular dyssynchrony,
139, 142
Inverted T waves
indication, 232
myocardial infarction,
195–196
myocardial ischaemia
LAD coronary artery,
193, 195
ST segment
depression, 193
Wellens' syndrome,
193–194
Isoelectric (normal) baseline,
166–167

J

Jervell and Lange–Nielsen
syndrome, 209

L

LAFB, *see* Left anterior fascicular
      block (LAFB)
LBBB, *see* Left bundle branch block
      (LBBB)
Left anterior descending (LAD)
      coronary artery,
      193, 195
Left anterior fascicular block
      (LAFB), 144–145
Left axis deviation
    angle, 21
    causes, 23
    left anterior fascicular
      block, 144
    QRS axis assessment, 22,
      223–224
Left bundle branch block (LBBB)
    causes, 139, 141
    CRT pacemaker, 139
    ECG in, 139–140
    interventricular
      dyssynchrony, 139
    pre-existing, 139, 141
    Purkinje fibres, 137
    QRS complex
      morphology, 120
    QRS complex shapes, 139
    Sgarbossa criteria, 141
Left posterior fascicular block
      (LPFB), 145–146, 230
Left ventricular aneurysm, 33,
      175–176

Left ventricular hypertrophy (LVH)
    ECG diagnosis, 154
    pressure overload, 154
    QRS complexes and, 230–231
    Sokolow–Lyon criteria, 154
    with strain, 156–157, 183
    tall R waves, 154–155
    voltage criteria, 154, 156
Long QT interval
    conditions, 210
    drugs and, 209–210
    in elderly patient, 211–212
    LQTS, 209
    polymorphic ventricular
      tachycardia, 207–208
    potassium/sodium channel
      problems, 209
    risk, 207–209
    TdP, 207–208
    treatment, 212
Long QT syndromes (LQTS),
      209, 212
Low-amplitude oscillations, 88–89
LPFB, *see* Left posterior fascicular
      block (LPFB)
LVH, *see* Left ventricular
      hypertrophy (LVH)

M

Maximum slope intercept method,
      QT interval, 200–201
Micro re-entry circuit, 103
Mobitz type I AV block,
      133, 134, 136

Mobitz type II AV block, 133, 135–136
Monomorphic ventricular tachycardia
  adult advanced life support algorithm, 116–117
  ARVC, 118
  atrioventricular dissociation, 119–120
  broad-complex tachycardia, 114–115, 119
  Brugada syndrome and, 118
  causes, 114, 116
  drug treatments, 116, 118
  ECG features, 120
  haemodynamic stability, 119
  idiopathic, 118
  management and correction, 116
  RVOT, 118
  symptoms, 116
Myocardial cells, 5–6, 221
Myocardial infarction; see also ST segment elevation myocardial infarction (STEMI)
  acute anterior, 190–191
  acute posterior, 181, 183–184
  inferior, 151–152
  QRS complex, 151–152
  ST segment, 165
  T waves changes,

Myocardial ischaemia
  depression, ST segment, 181–182
  heart rhythms, 67
  ST segment, 165
  T wave changes
    LAD coronary artery, 193, 195
    ST segment depression, 193
    Wellens' syndrome, 193–194
Myocytes, 5–7

N

Narrow-complex tachycardia, 57, 226
Non-ST segment elevation myocardial infarction (NSTEMI), 195

O

Orthodromic atrioventricular re-entry tachycardia (AVRT), 99, 101
Outpatient ECG monitoring
  cardiomemo devices, 216–217
  continuous ambulatory monitors, 216
  heart rhythm problems, 215–216
  implantable loop recorders (see Implantable ECG loop

P

Pacemaker
 AV junctional, 147
 backup, 146
 cells, 5, 221
 CRT, 139
 heart's natural, 6
 pacing 'on demand,' 163
 permanent, 86
 sinoatrial node, 9
 sinus rhythm, 79
 ventricular pacing, 161
Pericarditis, 177, 179–180
Polymorphic ventricular tachycardia
  categories, 124
  long QT interval, 207–208
  QRS complex morphology,
   124–125
  torsades de pointes, 124
  treatment, 124, 127
Posterior chest leads, ECG, 32–33
Premature atrial contractions
   (PACs), 86
Premature ventricular contractions
   (PVCs), 107
PR interval
 ECG, 18, 43, 222
 first-degree AV block, 130, 145
 second-degree AV block, 133
 short, 97, 99–100, 223
 supraventricular rhythms, 96
Prinzmetal's (vasospastic) angina,
   177–178, 231

Purkinje fibres
 electrical system, heart, 10, 222
 LBBB, 137
 RBBB, 142
P waves
 atrial activity, cardiac rhythm,
  74–75
 independent activity, 120–121
 rate, 52–53
 SA node, 130–131
 ventricular activity, cardiac
   rhythm, 69

Q

QRS (cardiac) axis
 complexes, 22–23
 depolarization waves, 19
 eyeball method, 22
 range of angles, 20–21
 ventricular depolarization,
   19–20
QRS complexes
 broad (see Broad QRS complex)
 counting
   automated heart rate
    calculations, 52
   ventricular rate calculation,
    50–51
 inferior myocardial infarction,
   151–152
 LVH, 154–156
 QRS axis, 22
 Q wave, 149, 151

RVH, 156, 158
septal depolarization, 149–150
small, 156, 159
ventricular rhythm, 69–70
QT interval
  correction
    Bazett's formula, 203–204
    'eyeball' approach, 205–206
    Fridericia's formula,
        203–204
    Hodges formula, 204
    QTc interval, 202
    smartphone apps, 205
  definition, 199, 232–233
  implantable cardioverter-
      defibrillator (ICD), 207
  long (see Long QT interval)
  measurement
    maximum slope intercept
        method, 200–201
    QRS complex, 200
    QRS duration, 201–202
    U waves, 200
  normal, 205
  risk, 207–208
  short, 207
Q wave, 149, 151

R

RBBB, see Right bundle branch
      block (RBBB)
Regular alarm noise, 215
Repolarization (early), ST segment

Resting heart rate, 17
Rhythm control, 90–91
Rhythm strip, 63–64
Right axis deviation, 23
Right bundle branch block (RBBB)
  causes, 141–142
  ECG features, 120
  interventricular
      dyssynchrony, 142
  QRS complexes, 142, 144
Right-sided chest leads, ECG,
      32–33, 35
Right ventricular hypertrophy
      (RVH), 156, 158
Right ventricular outflow tract
      (RVOT), 118
Romano–Ward syndrome, 209
R wave, 151, 154–155

S

Second-degree AV block
  AV conduction failure, 133
  bradycardia, 54
  Mobitz type I AV block,
      133–134
  Mobitz type II AV block,
      133, 135
  pacing in, 136
Shock, heart rhythms, 67
Short QT interval, 207
Sick sinus syndrome
  bradycardia, 54
  pacemaker, 86

in sinus arrest, 86
sinus node dysfunction, 84
tachycardia–bradycardia
syndrome, 86
Sinoatrial (SA) node
ECG waves, 14
electrical system, heart, 9
pacemaker cells, 5
problems (*see* Conduction
problems)
sick sinus syndrome, 86
Sinus arrhythmia
cardiac rhythms, 71
inspiration and expiration, 79, 82
physiological, 81
Sinus bradycardia
in bradycardic patient, 54–55
symptomatic, 82–83
Sinus rhythm, 79–80
Sinus tachycardia
narrow-complex
tachycardias, 57, 59
supraventricular
rhythms, 84–85
Skin preparation, 12-lead ECG
recording
chest hair removal, 26
cleansing, 27
light abrasion, 26
Society for Cardiological Science
and Technology, 25
STEMI, *see* ST segment elevation
myocardial infarction
(STEMI)

Stroke
risk reduction, 88, 90
volume, 3
ST segment
definition, 165
depression (*see* Depression, ST
segment)
elevation (*see* Elevation, ST
segment)
isoelectric (normal) baseline,
166–167
J point, 166, 168, 170
myocardial
infarction, 165
myocardial ischaemia, 165
ST segment elevation myocardial
infarction (STEMI)
acute coronary syndrome
(ACS), 170
anteroseptal, 173–174
Brugada syndrome, 170
clinical features, 170
contiguous leads, 171
coronary
revascularization, 173
differential diagnosis, 170
ECG leads and myocardial
territories, 171
high-risk acute coronary
syndromes, 173
inferior, 171–172
myocardial infarction, 195
posterior, 175

Supraventricular rhythms
    AF (*see* Atrial fibrillation (AF))
    atrial ectopic beats, 86–87
    atrial flutter (*see* Atrial flutter)
    atrial tachycardia, 94–95
    AVNRT (*see* AV nodal re-entry
        tachycardia (AVNRT))
    AVRT (*see* AV re-entry
        tachycardia (AVRT))
    features, 228
    His–Purkinje system, 102
    PR interval, 96
    sick sinus syndrome
        pacemaker, 86
        in SA block, 86
        in sinus arrest, 86
        sinus node dysfunction, 84
        tachycardia–bradycardia
          syndrome, 86
    sinus arrhythmia, 79, 81–82
    sinus bradycardia, 82–83
    sinus rhythm, 79–80
    sinus tachycardia, 84–85
Supraventricular tachycardias
    (SVTs), 60–61, 227
S wave, 151
Syncope, 67, 116
Systole, 1, 4, 221

T

Tachycardia; *see also* Heart rate
    adult tachycardia
        algorithm, 60–61

    causes, 226–227
    definition, 17, 52, 57
    identification, 57
    management, 61
    narrow-complex, 57, 61
    sinus tachycardia, 57, 59
    SVTs, 61
    ventricular fibrillation, 61
Tachycardia–bradycardia
        syndrome, 86
Third-degree AV block
    AV conduction, 136, 138
    bradycardia, 54
    causes, 136–137
    conduction interruption, 136
Three-electrode ECG, 213–214
Torsades de pointes (TdP),
        207–208
Trifascicular block, 145
T waves changes
    acute anterior myocardial
        infarction, 190–191
    hyperkalaemia, 187, 189–190
    hypokalaemia, 190, 192
    hypothyroidism, 190
    indication, 232
    myocardial infarction,
        195–196
    myocardial ischaemia
        LAD coronary artery,
          193, 195
        ST segment depression, 193
        Wellens' syndrome,
          193, 194

STEMI, 190–191
ventricles repolarization, 232
Wellens' syndrome, 193–194
12-lead ECG reading
    clinical data, 42
    comprehensive ECG
        report, 44–45
    fundamental features,
        43, 225–226
    patient data, 41
    technical data, 42
12-lead ECG recording
    in dextrocardia, 34
    electrode placement
        chest (precordial)
            electrodes, 28, 30–31
        colour codes, 27
        in female patients, 31
        limb electrodes, 28
        misplacement, 28
        parts, 27
        "Ride Your Green
            Bike", 28
    electronic patient record, 34
    errors, 25
    paper speed and gain
        settings, 36–37
    patient encourage, 35
    preparations, 25–26, 224
    skin preparation, 26–27
    special electrode
        positions, 32–33
    standard settings, 36

U

U waves, 192, 200

V

Valsalva manoeuvre, 102–103
VEBs, see Ventricular ectopic
        beats (VEBs)
Ventricular activity, cardiac
        rhythm
    asystole, 67–68
    atrial activity, 75–76
    broad-complex vs. narrow-
        complex rhythms, 74
    His–Purkinje system, 72–73
    P waves, 69
    QRS complexes, 67, 70, 72–73
    regular/irregular, 69–70
    ventricular ectopic beat, 73
    ventricular rate, 69
Ventricular bigeminy, 108, 110
Ventricular couplet, 111
Ventricular ectopic beats (VEBs)
    causes, 107–108
    electrophysiological
        ablation, 111
    fatal arrhythmias, 111
    multifocal, 108
    multiple, 108
    occurrence, 108–109
    R on T, 111–112
    T wave and, 195
    unifocal, 108

Ventricular extrasystoles, 107
Ventricular fibrillation
    cardiac arrest rhythm, 61
    causes, 127
    chaotic rhythm, 126–127
Ventricular pacing, 161–162
Ventricular pre-excitation, 97–98
Ventricular premature beats
      (VPBs), 107
Ventricular premature complexes
      (VPCs), 107
Ventricular quadrigeminy, 108
Ventricular rate, 47, 90
Ventricular rhythms
    broad-complex tachycardia, 229
    cardiac rhythm, 69–70
    idioventricular rhythm
        (see Accelerated
        idioventricular rhythm)
    monomorphic ventricular
        tachycardia (see
        Monomorphic
        ventricular tachycardia)
    polymorphic ventricular
        tachycardia
        categories, 124
        QRS complex morphology,
          124–125
        torsades de
          pointes, 124
        treatment, 124, 127
    VEBs (see Ventricular ectopic
        beats (VEBs))
    ventricular fibrillation,
        126–127, 229
Ventricular systole and
      diastole, 3–4
Ventricular tachycardia, 111
Ventricular trigeminy, 108

W

Wellens' syndrome, 193–194
Wolff–Parkinson–White
      (WPW) syndrome,
      23, 99, 102

T - #0043 - 161024 - C272 - 144/104/13 - PB - 9781498705936 - Gloss Lamination